The Cardiac Recovery Handbook

The Cardiac Recovery Handbook

The Complete Guide to Life after Heart Attack or Heart Surgery

Paul Kligfield, MD
and Michelle D. Seaton

with an Afterword by Frederic Flach, MD, KCHS

healthyliving**books**

New York

Figures on pages 47, 48, 65, 104, 122 reprinted from *Textbook of Medical Physiology,* 10th edition, Arthur C. Guyton M.D. and John E. Hall, pages 97, 226, 232, 280, 698, Copyright 2000, with permission from Elsevier.

Figures on page 53 reprinted from the *New England Journal of Medicine,* Vol. 340 No. 2, Russel Ross, Ph.D., "Atherosclerosis—An Inflammatory Disease," pages 117, 118, Copyright 1999 Massachusetts Medical Society. All rights reserved.

Figure on page 124 reprinted from the *American Journal of Medicine,* Vol. 112 (2), Amir Halkin, M.D. & Gad Keren, M.D., "Potential indications for angiotensin-converting enzyme inhibitors in atherosclerotic vascular disease," page 127, Copyright 2002, with permission from Excerpta Medica Inc.

This book does not give legal or medical advice. Always consult your lawyer, doctor, and other professionals. The names of people who contributed anecdotal material have been changed. The ideas and suggestions contained in this book are not intended as a substitute for consulting with a physician. All matters regarding your health require medical supervision.

This edition is printed on acid-free paper that meets the American National Standards Institute Z39-48 Standard.

Library of Congress Cataloging-in-Publication Data

Kligfield, Paul.
    The cardiac recovery handbook : the complete guide to life after heart attack or heart surgery/ Paul Kligfield and Michelle Seaton.
       p. cm.
    ISBN 1-57826-142-2 (hardcover : alk. paper)
    1. Myocardial infarction--Popular works. 2. Heart--Surgery--Popular works. I. Seaton, Michelle. II. Title.
    RC685.I6K54 2004
    616.1'23706--dc22

                              2003026655

All Hatherleigh Press titles are available for bulk purchase, special promotions, and premiums. For more information, please contact the manager of our Special Sales Department at 1-800-528-2550.

Healthy Living Books
Hatherleigh Press
5-22 46th Avenue, Suite 200
Long Island City, NY 11101
1-800-528-2550

Designed by Tai Blanche

Printed in Canada

10 9 8 7 6 5 4 3 2 1

♦ ♦ ❖ ♦ ♦ ♦ ❖ ♦ ♦ ❖ ♦ ♦ ❖ ♦ ♦ ❖ ♦ ♦ ❖ ♦ ♦

For Mary and Ben, with love; for the magnificent staff at the Cardiac
Health Center, with thanks; for investigators in cardiovascular
medicine and surgery, with appreciation; and for patients with heart
disease, who have taught me so much.

Contents

◆ ◆ ❖ ◆ ◆ ❖ ◆ ◆ ❖ ◆ ◆ ❖ ◆ ◆ ❖ ◆ ◆ ❖ ◆ ◆

Introduction

◆ ◆ ❖ ◆ ◆ ❖ ◆ ◆ ❖ ◆ ◆ ❖ ◆ ◆ ❖ ◆ ◆ ❖ ◆ ◆

When I see patients after their heart attack, angioplasty, or bypass surgery, I know that they are full of uncertainty and fear about their future. Many patients come to these appointments still shaken by the pain and helplessness they felt during their heart attack and hospital stay. The reality—and it is a reality—that having coronary artery disease puts you at increased risk for suffering a potentially fatal heart attack in the future only compounds that fear. But the good news is that the medical progress of the past few decades has dramatically improved the outlook for most patients with heart disease. This book will help you to gain confidence and to reduce your risk of future cardiac problems.

I believe that my role in the care of patients with heart disease is not simply to administer tests, write prescriptions, and anticipate problems, but also to educate them about the ways in which heart and arterial disease affect the body and how medication and lifestyle choices can favorably alter the course of the disease. Patients who understand the nature of heart disease improve not only their chances for survival but also their quality of life. Knowledge is empowering. I believe that the more you know about your disease and its management, the better able you will be to work with your own doctor for a successful long-term recovery.

So, if you have recently survived a heart attack, needed bypass surgery or angioplasty, or have chest pain due to coronary disease, this book is for you. I wrote *The Cardiac Recovery Handbook* as a way to help guide you to a longer, more comfortable, and more active life.

You'll learn about the medications you have been prescribed, why they are useful, how they affect your body, and how they can reduce your risk of future complications from heart disease. In addition, the book will take you through the many important choices you make every day that can either help or hinder your progress.

The first thing you'll want to do is take stock of where you are and what has happened to you in the hospital. Part I of this book addresses those issues as well as the transition you face when you come home from the hospital. Chapter 3 highlights the incredible advances made in the study of heart disease in the past half century. I think many people will be reassured by the dramatic improvements in the outcome of heart disease in our lifetime: Mortality and disability have been significantly reduced to improve recovery. You will learn about the causes of arterial disease and the risk factors that accelerate the development of arterial plaque. This is necessary in order to understand the medication and lifestyle changes that can reduce your risk of further coronary events.

If you have recently been diagnosed with heart disease, you have probably been given what seems like a lot of pills to take. No one likes to take medication on a long-term basis, and it is clear that many patients do not always take what is prescribed for them. Some of this is explained by the cost of medication, but much is due to a lack of real understanding of what these medications actually do, and precisely how and why they reduce risk. In the second part of the book, you'll read about four classes of medications commonly prescribed to heart patients. Once you understand the rationale for each medication, you can ask: If I am taking this drug, why am I taking it, and if not, why not? You can also better anticipate side effects and complications of these medications.

The third part of the book examines other critical elements of risk factor reduction, such as beginning an exercise program, losing weight, and quitting smoking. For example, many cardiac patients are afraid to exercise, while others don't believe that exercise really reduces the risk of developing heart disease. Actually, exercise has a stunning effect on nearly every aspect of heart disease, from its symptoms to its underlying pathology—regardless of your age. There is also a chapter in this section on emotional risk factors, such as stress, depression, and hostility. Unfortunately, depression and stress exacerbate arterial disease, and equally unfortunately, heart attack or heart surgery can trigger depression and stress. A final chapter will help you to understand the link between your emotions and your health and give you some guidelines for breaking the cycle.

The medications and lifestyle choices—called interventions—described in Part II and Part III of this book are not new ideas. These measures are strongly endorsed and promoted by major health organizations, including the American Heart Association and the American College of Cardiology. These interventions are not speculative or based solely on theory—they have been shown to improve survival in carefully performed clinical trials involving large groups of patients. In many cases, I've included details on some of these studies because the results are both encouraging and quite remarkable.

At the end of every chapter, I've included a list of pertinent questions for you to consider or to take to your next doctor's appointment. A concise definition of terms can be found in the Glossary in Appendix II.

My best general advice to anyone with heart disease is to understand what you should be doing to optimize your recovery and figure out whether you are doing things right. This includes maximizing office visits with your doctor by preparing questions about your treatment. The diagnosis of heart disease is often an emotionally overwhelming experience and the treatments available are somewhat complicated, particularly when the explanations are clouded by clinical jargon. Ideally, this book will help clarify some of the information your doctor has given you and at the same time spark questions about your treatment options. It is my hope that this book can be an ongoing resource to help you fully participate in your own recovery and good health.

◆ ◆ ❖ ◆ ◆ ❖ ◆ ◆ ❖ ◆ ◆ ❖ ◆ ◆ ❖ ◆ ◆ ❖ ◆ ◆ ❖ ◆ ◆ ❖ ◆ ◆ ❖

Decades ago, people feared heart disease—and with good reason—because doctors knew so little about how to prevent and treat heart attacks and coronary artery disease. It is natural to fear something that you can't understand, particularly when you can't control it. Today, doctors and researchers know a lot about what causes heart disease and how it affects the body. More important, there have been tremendous advances in treatment of heart disease. In fact, the death rate from heart disease in the United States has decreased markedly over the past 40 years.

Because of medical progress, heart disease now is more of a chronic condition—one that is managed with medication and lifestyle choices. Heart disease and its consequences are now generally understandable and treatable, and you have access to information that bears on your health.

The first thing information can do is improve your confidence, because, in general, the outlook for patients with most forms of heart

PART I

◆ ◆ ❖ ◆ ◆ ❖ ◆ ◆ ❖ ◆ ◆ ❖ ◆ ◆ ❖ ◆ ◆ ❖ ◆ ◆ ❖ ◆ ◆ ❖ ◆ ◆

Understanding Heart Disease

disease is good. Confidence also comes from knowledge. The more you know about the way your heart works and the role of coronary blood supply in the nutrition of your heart, the better you will understand how certain tests and revascularization procedures work. The more you know about risk factors and their consequences, the more motivated and better prepared you will be to change them to improve your health. The more you know about medications your doctor may ask you to take, the more likely you are to appreciate their importance, remember to take them, and report any side effects they may cause.

This book is designed to give a basic grounding in all of these areas. Since every patient is different, this cannot be a comprehensive discussion of your individual condition. Instead, it is intended as a guide to help you fill in some of the gaps in your information and ask better questions of your doctor.

Chapter 1

◆ ◆ ❖ ◆ ◆ ❖ ◆ ◆ ❖ ◆ ◆ ❖ ◆ ◆ ❖ ◆ ◆ ❖ ◆ ◆

The Diagnosis Is Heart Disease
What Happened in the Hospital

The diagnosis of heart disease is a life-altering event, but heart disease is a condition that can be managed with testing, treatments, lifestyle changes, and medication. Before you can consider these possibilities, you'll have to confront the physical and emotional effects of your diagnosis.

In this chapter, you'll read about the different emergency treatments you may have undergone in the hospital, including angioplasty, stenting, and bypass surgery. You'll also learn about the difference between *primary* prevention (the advice your doctor was giving you before your hospitalization) and *secondary* prevention (the advice your doctor will likely give you now). Finally, you'll learn about the issues involved in managing your heart disease long-term.

Your Experience of Heart Disease

Four years ago in January, I was at our annual office party. I was the emcee and I guess I had a heart attack. I don't remember anything from about 1:00 that afternoon on. Everything I know about that day, and that night and the following week, really, is what was told to me.
David K.

> *My husband was introducing people at the party. I turned to say*
> *something to someone next to me and when I turned back, he was*
> *gone. The fireman sitting at our table went up to where he had*
> *fallen and a nurse came up from the back of the room. They did two-*
> *man CPR on him for 25 minutes. We live in a fairly small town,*
> *and it was a Saturday night, so they had only one person on call.*
> *When the ambulance finally arrived, I wasn't feeling too good, so*
> *they brought an ambulance for me, too. They thought I was having*
> *a heart attack and wanted to admit me to the hospital.*
> *Lynn K., wife of David K.*

You may have realized that you have heart disease only after waking up in a hospital room following a heart attack with little or no memory of the events that brought you there. You may even have had an emergency angioplasty or emergency heart surgery without remembering it. The first days—and even weeks—following hospitalization for serious heart disease can be physically and emotionally overwhelming for you, the patient, as well as your family.

Recovery means healing from a heart attack, from surgery or other procedures, as well as getting used to a new set of physical sensations and adjusting to a host of new medications. Under these conditions, you may be so focused on the moment-to-moment activities associated with leaving the hospital and resuming your daily activities, that you may not have the energy or ability to ask important questions about what you can do to improve your long-term health and prevent another heart emergency.

Maybe you've had only a mild heart attack and have been lucky enough to avoid serious heart damage. Maybe you have just recently been diagnosed with angina due to coronary artery disease. Or, you may be one of the many people who arrive at a diagnosis of heart disease after a careful evaluation of symptoms, such as chest pain or shortness of breath, identified by a stress test, echocardiograph, or angiogram. For many people, the first symptoms of heart disease come in the form of a near-fatal heart attack.

They told me that the EMTs hit me with the paddles right there in the restaurant, and again when we got to the hospital. The doctor was waiting for me at the hospital and started asking for all these medicines, but the hospital didn't carry some of them. They had to send to another town for them, and the doctor decided to send me to the heart center in Lincoln, Nebraska, which is 100 miles away. They put me back in an ambulance and the doctor said to the driver, "Don't stop for anything." I guess we got to Lincoln in a little over an hour. My son told me that when they took me out of the ambulance, it took four nurses to subdue me. I kept trying to yank off the ventilator and IVs and get out of there.
David K.

By the time I got to the heart center in Lincoln, David was unconscious and in the ICU. Still, they had him strapped down because he had been so combative. That bothered me. He was sedated until Monday. On Tuesday he had an angiogram, and it showed three blocked arteries. He needed a triple bypass, and he needed it the next day. The following Tuesday they sent him home. I remember him getting out of the ambulance. He was so pale, and I was thinking that he'd had all of this medical attention to save his life, and here he is at home. I was thinking, "What am I supposed to do with him? What if something goes wrong?"
Lynn K.

If you are reading this book, you probably have your own story—uncomfortable symptoms, a failed stress test, a cardiac catheterization, or a heart attack. Your doctor may have told you that you have heart disease and referred you to a heart specialist, known as a cardiologist. By this point, you are probably wondering what you need to do to minimize your complications, improve your health, and start to feel better about your condition.

What Recovery Means

Although there are many approaches to recovery, a good beginning is to get information about heart disease, including understanding the lifestyle choices and other risk factors that have contributed to it. You will want find out about what tests are used to evaluate your progress and what the results mean. You'll also want to learn about the various treatment options, including medications and procedures. You will want to understand why treatment is effective and how much difference appropriate treatment can make in your future. When people have difficulty with their care, it is often because they fail to do one or more of the following things:

* *Understand the nature of heart disease and the importance of participating in your own care.*

* *Make lifestyle changes that can reduce the risk of having another heart attack or coronary event.*

* *Take prescribed medications that can reduce symptoms and improve survival.*

* *Make important follow-up appointments with your cardiologist to test and track your progress.*

What Happened in the Hospital?

If your symptoms required a stay in the hospital or if you needed to have an emergency procedure or surgery, you need to understand what has happened to you before you can cope with the ongoing management of your condition. That's quite normal.

There is no typical hospital experience for people with heart disease. The care you received was tailored to your individual case. Exactly what kind of treatments and medications a person receives depends on a number of factors. For example, you may have been admitted to the hospital because:

* *Your doctor ordered elective tests to diagnose and treat chest pain (angina) that you were having as a result of obstructions in the coronary arteries that feed the heart.*

* *Your symptoms of angina were becoming more severe or more frequent, or could be precipitated by less and less exercise. Doctors refer to this as unstable or crescendo angina.*

* *You were admitted to the emergency room with sustained chest discomfort, persistent even at rest, due to severe blockages in*

one or more coronary arteries. *This is much more serious than the temporary discomfort of exercise-related angina because these blockages are likely to cause actual damage to the pumping muscles of your heart. Blood tests and an electrocardiogram are used to track the evolving nature of this damage, known as a myocardial infarction (or more commonly as a heart attack). The more damage the heart muscle suffers, the more severe the heart attack is considered.*

★ *You were rushed to the hospital after a catastrophic collapse caused by a serious rhythm irregularity of the heart. This can occur during the early course of a heart attack.*

Whatever the reason for admission, you would have received a number of treatments and you will have undergone one or more diagnostic or therapeutic procedures. These might include medications, such as blood thinners and anti-clotting drugs, as well as nitroglycerine to dilate the arteries. You also may have received drugs such as beta-blockers that reduce the work of the heart, anti-cholesterol medications, one or more medications to lower your blood pressure, along with further adjustments of your regular medicine.

Non-Emergency Hospitalization

Twelve years ago I was short of breath during a walk. A friend who was walking with me wondered why I was huffing and puffing. He told me to get to a doctor for a stress test, which I did the next day. During the test, the doctor told me to get off the treadmill. "This doesn't look good," he said. And he told me to see a cardiologist.
Samuel S.

If your doctor admitted you to the hospital for testing, usually for suspected stable or unstable angina, your diagnosis may have started with an exercise test, which led to a coronary *angiogram*. This is a procedure that allows the blood flow in the coronary arteries to be filmed and analyzed. If this revealed one or more serious obstructions that were related to your symptoms, you may have received a coronary *angioplasty* to open the blocked artery.

Heart Attack

I had what doctors told me was a heart attack in 1985. I'd had symptoms and I dropped by my doctor's office when I could work it into my schedule. I told him my symptoms, and he did an ECG and said, "You've had a heart attack. You have to go to the hospital." I told him I had to go home first, and he said, "You don't understand. You're going right now." He put me in a cab to New York Hospital and I was there for a week.
Donald D.

The diagnosis of a heart attack is made from the symptoms, the electrocardiogram, and blood tests taken during your initial evaluation. The severity of changes in the ECG and blood test abnormalities often, but not always, reflects the severity of the ongoing heart muscle damage.

If you were admitted to the hospital early in the course of your heart attack, the doctors in the emergency room would have tried to limit the damage to the heart muscle by getting rid of the clot in the artery that was causing the heart attack. Depending on the severity of your situation and the availability of different procedures in your community, you may have been treated with medication to dissolve the clot or you may have been rushed to the catheterization laboratory for angiography, possibly followed by angioplasty and stenting to open the artery.

After the blockages had been removed, you would have been observed more carefully for several more days. You would have begun walking as soon as you were able, and you would have been encouraged to walk more each day to allow the heart to begin its healing process. If a heart attack led to angioplasty or surgical bypass, your discharge would have been governed by your individual ability to heal.

Blood Tests for Heart Attacks

I was on vacation, doing some skeet shooting at a big resort and I started sweating profusely, and I got sick to my stomach. I also got a strange feeling in my arm, not a pain, there was never any pain, but I felt weak. I went to the little clinic there and they did some blood tests. Those tests found some enzymes showing heart damage. That's how I knew I had a heart attack.
Demetre S.

If you go to the hospital because you think you are having a heart attack, one of the first things doctors will do is a blood test.

A heart attack is a condition in which the cells in your heart are so starved for oxygen that they begin to die. As they do, they release chemicals that circulate in the blood. These chemicals include:

Creatine Kinase (CK-MB). One form of creatine kinase, known as the MB form, is a fairly reliable marker for heart injury. The level of CK-MB rises within 3–12 hours of a heart attack. It generally peaks in 24 hours and then returns to normal. The trouble is that some other types of cells also release CK-MB when they have suffered damage. Surgery, injury, and some diseases can also increase the level of CK-MB in your blood.

Cardiac-Specific Troponin T and Troponin I. These are the most sensitive cardiac markers, and they are able to identify even very slight damage to myocardial cells. Unlike CK, they are almost never present in the blood, except in some patients with kidney disease, unless you are having a heart attack. Plus, the troponin markers can circulate in the blood for up to 5–10 days after the first symptoms of a heart attack, making diagnosis possible even after the heart attack has ended.

Other Cardiac Muscle Enzymes. There are other cardiac muscle enzymes that are released from injured heart muscles, and these can be useful for diagnosis under some circumstances. These include enzymes known as SGOT and LDH, and a delayed appearance and disappearance of LDH relative to SGOT in the years prior to more widespread use of troponin and CK was considered to be characteristic of recent infarction. However, other tissues such as the liver also contain these enzymes, which makes troponin and CK the more commonly used markers.

Angioplasty with Stent

I had a heart attack in May, 2001, and had an angioplasty after and they put a stent in. A day and a half later, I had pains again. And they had to go back in and put in another stent. The scar tissue had closed it up.
Jeff G.

Angioplasty is a procedure that involves opening the artery by inflating a balloon at the end of a specialized catheter during a catheterization. It is considered less invasive than bypass surgery because it can be performed using mild sedation and local anesthesia at the site, generally in the groin, where the catheter is introduced. It sometimes includes placing a tiny mesh tube, called a *stent,* in the artery at the site of the blockage to help to prevent the artery from closing up again.

If you had an angioplasty procedure because of stable or unstable angina, and suffered no damage to the heart, you would have been walking actively by the next day, and your doctor would have discharged you from the hospital as soon as your condition was stable.

Bypass Surgery

After my surgery, the physical recovery was difficult. They break open your chest and put it back together. There was a lot of pain. I had a quadruple bypass, but it doesn't make any difference. You go through bypass, they are still opening the chest.
Ivan B.

After my bypass surgery, I loved going to bed each night, because I knew I would feel so much better the next morning. You improve so quickly.
Donald D.

If the obstructions in your arteries were so severe that the likelihood of successful angioplasty and stenting was in doubt, you may have undergone coronary artery *bypass surgery.* This is a major operation in which blood flow is routed around the clogged coronary arteries by

What Happened in the ER?

If you were taken to the hospital emergency room with heart attack symptoms, there was probably a flurry of activity. All of this was designed to diagnose the problem immediately and begin treatment to prevent or minimize long-term complications. Treatments generally include:

* *A physical assessment, including vital signs and estimation of blood oxygen levels.*

* *Supplemental oxygen, if needed.*

* *Nitroglycerin to dilate the blood vessels, improve blood flow, and decrease pain. This can be administered in tablet-form under the tongue every five minutes or intravenously.*

* *Pain medication, if needed.*

* *A blood test to look for substances that are released into the blood during a heart attack, called serum cardiac markers.*

* *Continuous ECG to monitor the heart's electrical activity to watch for serious abnormalities of rhythm.*

* *In addition, a standard ECG will be done to give clues as to the presence, type, and location of arterial blockage the heart has suffered.*

* *A dose of aspirin to decrease the aggregation ("stickiness") of blood platelets and to help prevent future blood clots, or another antiplatelet agent, or maybe both.*

* *A beta-blocker to reduce the workload of the heart, decrease the damage to the heart muscle, and decrease the chances that the heart will develop ventricular arrhythmias that can lead to fibrillation.*

* *A dose of a statin drug, used for lowering cholesterol. In the midst of a heart attack, these drugs may also help to stabilize coronary plaque.*

In addition to all of this, doctors will consider other procedures or medications to improve blood flow through the blocked coronary arteries. Depending on the kind of heart attack, its location, and the facilities available at the treating facility, this might include:

* *Drugs that modify the blood clotting system*

* *"Clot-busting" drugs to dissolve blockages*

* *Immediate angioplasty with stenting to open the artery*

* *Emergency bypass surgery (rarely)*

The decision on whether and how to carry out revascularization needs to be made quickly for the best outcome.

attaching a piece of blood vessel taken from another part of the body to create a detour for the coronary circulation.

Coronary artery bypass surgery (CABG) uses veins (usually from the legs) or arteries (from the chest wall or arm) to go around the obstructions in the coronary arteries. This is generally done under heart bypass, a procedure in which the blood and oxygen flow to the body is controlled by a mechanical pump-oxygenator.

The standard surgical incision for this procedure is to open the breastbone down the middle. Sometimes the operation can be done by accessing the heart through the ribs on one side of the chest. And more recently, bypass surgery can sometimes be performed through a relatively small incision on the chest wall, sparing the need to cut through the breast bone. At times, it is even possible to operate on the beating heart, which avoids the complications of the heart bypass pump. However, for most people, bypass surgery is still an open-heart operation that requires the larger incision. So if you had bypass surgery, you probably will have a fairly big scar down the center of your chest, along with scars on one or both thighs where veins were harvested for use as bypass vessels by the surgeon.

Immediately after bypass surgery, you may remember having a breathing tube temporarily in place while you regained strength and consciousness after anesthesia. You also had one or more chest tubes to drain blood and other fluids from the outside linings of the heart and lungs. Pacemaker wires may have been left on the surface of the heart to control any rhythm irregularities after surgery; these wires and tubes would have been removed after a few days.

Many people have remarkably little physical pain after bypass surgery. Some even report greater discomfort at the site of the leg incision than the chest incision. Other patients have chest pain after surgery, which can last, usually in mild form, for several months. A few people experience a nagging pain that may last for many months, or, rarely, up to a year. This pain is markedly different from angina, and is caused by the wound as it knits together. If you had a mammary artery harvested for use in the bypass surgery, you will have an additional wound inside the chest wall where the artery was removed.

Heart Attack Prevention

> *I advise people now who are nearing 60; I had my first event at 59. I tell people who are that age, if you have any kind of disturbance, go to a cardiologist. Just from so many people having different symptoms.*
> *Dennis L.*

The management of heart disease, which is an attempt to prevent a heart attack or other complications, can be separated into the following three phases.

Primary prevention. Primary care physicians provide education to people who don't yet have heart disease but may have risk factors for the development of atherosclerosis. The goal is to modify risk factors and prevent a first heart attack, stroke, or diagnosis of heart disease. Unfortunately, individuals who don't see a primary care physician for routine checkups have no reliable way of effectively acting on current information about their own health or their risk factors.

The Role of Pacemakers and Implantable Defibrillators

I needed a pacemaker because my heart rate had become so low. I was having episodes of dizziness and weakness. When I went to the hospital, my heart rate was down to 37. I had a pacer put in last summer, and I did not feel well at all afterward. If anything I had worse symptoms. Shortness of breath, dizziness, weakness. After three weeks they determined that one lead was not in the right place. They shut down the one lead, then had the surgery redone. It was better but not great. The doctor finally determined that my natural pacemaker was fighting with the new pacemaker, so they decided to slow down my natural heartbeat with medication and let the new pacemaker take over. Things have started to get better in the last month or so.
Helen S.

Many people are familiar with the type of pacemaker used to regulate heart rates that have become too slow. However, there are two new types of pacemakers that can help patients with heart failure. It is important to note that these are not suitable for everyone, and doctors are still working to establish the best criteria for selecting appropriate patients.

One of these pacemakers, known as the implantable pacemaker-defibrillator, keeps track of the heart rhythm and delivers an electrical shock to the heart if a potentially lethal ventricular rhythm, such as ventricular tachycardia or ventricular fibrillation, develops. With this device, you are, in effect, carrying your own internally implanted heart defibrillator around with you. You may want to ask your doctor about this device if you have heart failure along with serious rhythm abnormalities.

A second new device that appears useful for some patients with heart failure is the biventricular pacemaker. Standard pacemakers stimulate the heart via a wire placed in the right ventricle. This creates an abnormal electrical pattern in the heart that sometimes results in reduced pumping power. The biventricular pacemaker uses synchronized pacing of the heart by two separate wires—one to each ventricle—to better simulate the heart's normal electrical activity. In some cases of heart failure, this can markedly improve heart performance.

Acute intervention. This phase often takes place in an ambulance, emergency room, coronary care unit, catheterization laboratory, or operating room when a patient is admitted with heart disease. The problem could be angina, unstable angina or a suspected heart attack, or the intervention could result from routine diagnostic testing. This phase includes interventions such as administration of thrombolytic (clot-dissolving) drugs, other intravenous drugs, diagnostic catheterization, angioplasty and stenting, and even open-heart surgery.

Some people take the step of contacting a cardiologist because they suspect that they have heart disease and they want to confirm this diagnosis. For these patients, acute intervention involves conducting tests, reducing symptoms, and modifying risk factors. These patients get a head start on the next phase of managing their disease, because they didn't wait for the heart attack to happen.

Secondary prevention. Once you've had the first cardiovascular event, it is evident that you suffer from cardiovascular disease. Further prevention becomes secondary rather than primary. Secondary prevention means that you work directly with a cardiologist or primary care physician to manage your symptoms and modify your risk factors to reduce the likelihood that a heart attack or stroke will ever happen again. This phase also includes regular appointments and testing to check your progress and monitor your body's reaction to any medications you may be taking.

Controlling Heart Disease Long-Term

Before my bypass surgery, I walked outside my hospital room and looked at the Atlantic Ocean, and I remember thinking, "I don't know if I'm ever going to see this ocean again." Afterward, I deliberately walked out and looked at it again. There is a certain amount of gratitude afterward, and then you get on this trip and you tell yourself you're going to do

everything, you're going to be so good, because this is never going to hap-
pen to me again. And then as humans we give up on it. We forget the
pain we were in.
Lou S.

The goal of secondary prevention is to prevent additional coronary events and the complications of heart disease. The best way to do this is to educate yourself about the interventions, meaning lifestyle changes and medications that can help you reduce your risk factors and to discuss these interventions with your doctor. This book is focused on the secondary interventions that have been shown in carefully designed scientific studies to improve survival and quality of life for patients with heart disease. Some, but not all, of these interventions are also important for primary prevention.

If you have been in the hospital with unstable angina or a heart attack, you have probably been given what may seem like a lot of different pills. No one likes to take medications, and it is reasonable to wonder: Are all these pills necessary? Are some more important than others? Other interventions may be inconvenient, or time consuming, and you will probably question why they are being recommended. Ultimately, the success of your treatment program depends on you and your doctor, and the support of your family. But the more you know about the reasons for medical and life style interventions, the better your decision process can be.

The rest of this book explains the nature of heart disease. It also describes currently accepted interventions and how they can dramatically reduce your chances of experiencing another coronary event. These interventions include:

* *Taking aspirin and other anti-coagulants*
* *Taking beta-blockers to alter the adrenaline response of the body*

* *Taking medications such as ACE inhibitors to regulate other aspects of the body response to stress*
* *Taking medications such as statins to help control cholesterol levels*
* *Participating in cardiac rehabilitation and increasing regular exercise*
* *Quitting smoking*
* *Controlling blood pressure*
* *Controlling diabetes*
* *Controlling diet and weight*
* *Dealing with stress, hostility, and depression*

Some Questions to Ask

For many people, the diagnosis of heart disease comes as the result of a stay in the hospital to receive urgent care for an episode of angina, treatment of a heart attack, or a surgical procedure such as angioplasty or bypass surgery. In the months ahead, you will want to learn as much as you can about heart disease and how you can prevent a future heart attack or surgery. But first you will want to ground yourself emotionally and come to terms with what happened to you in the hospital. This may involve piecing together events that you may not remember clearly. Some questions you can ask your doctor and family members include:

* *Why was I hospitalized?*
* *What happened to me in the hospital? What treatments and medications was I given?*
* *Did I have a heart attack? Did I suffer damage to the heart muscle?*
* *Given my age and general health, what length of recovery can I expect?*
* *What kind of pain or other physical sensations can I expect? What side effects are common for the medications I'll be taking?*

* *When can I resume my normal activities? When can I drive? When can I go back to work? When can I travel?*

* *What kinds of follow-up appointments should I schedule to check my surgical wounds or to take blood tests to make sure my medications are working?*

* *Can my primary care physician manage my heart disease or should I look for a cardiologist?*

Chapter 2

❖ ❖ ❖ ❖ ❖ ❖ ❖ ❖ ❖ ❖ ❖ ❖ ❖ ❖ ❖ ❖ ❖ ❖ ❖

First Steps in Your Cardiac Recovery

What Happens When You Get Home

In the weeks after emergency surgery or angioplasty, you'll need some guidelines for making the transition from hospital to home and advice for finding a cardiologist you trust, someone who will answer your questions and recommend appropriate treatments. In this chapter, you will read about what to expect during the first weeks and months of recovery. You'll also get advice about how to adapt to new symptoms and physical sensations, and you'll read guidelines for when to seek emergency medical attention.

> *The doctor kept me in the hospital for a day after they put the stent in. Then he made me stay home for a few more days after I got home before I could return to work. Considering that I had a heart attack, the recovery wasn't as big a deal as I thought it would be.*
> *Margaret G.*

> *The last question I asked my doctor after my bypass was "When can I have sex?" The doctor said, "When you can climb a flight of stairs." I said, "What do I get for a couple of steps?"*
> *Dennis L.*

What being home again is like will obviously depend on what your condition was and the treatments you received for it. For example:

An episode of angina. If your angina has responded to medication, you will find you have more tolerance for exercise. Since you didn't experience any heart muscle damage, you will not need a specific recovery period and can generally resume your regular activities as your doctor allows. Obviously, you will want to be sure that you are doing everything you can to minimize the risk of additional coronary disease.

Angioplasty with stent. If you have had a stent inserted, you will need to take a drug to prevent blood clots from forming inside the stent in addition to your regular medications. You may need take the drug for only a limited period, such as a month, or you may need to continue it indefinitely. In addition to clots inside the stent, abnormal growth of the arterial wall around the stent can cause stents to close. The risk of a stent closing up after implantation has been markedly decreased by a coating of medication on some stents that reduce the overgrowth of muscle that leads to the production of scar tissue around the stent. Your cardiologist will probably want to see you for a follow-up visit to check the progress of your healing at the site where the catheter was inserted, and to check for any other complications.

Some doctors and researchers have suggested that heavy physical exertion can cause blood clots to develop within stents in the few weeks after implantation. The validity of these observations is arguable, but still it is likely that after stent implantation, your cardiologist may recommend that you avoid extreme physical activity for about a month. Implanting a stent does cause some trauma to the inner lining of the artery, and the body's primary response to trauma is to create blood clots to stop bleeding and scar tissue to heal the injury. In the short term, heavy physical exertion and the adrenaline that comes with it may further injure the area around the stent and encourage more blood clots.

However, after this period has passed, a regular program of exercise is as important as anything else you can do to protect the stent and to reduce your risk of further cardiac events. Over time, regular exercise will actually help the artery to relax, and will make the artery more resistant to the irritating effects of adrenaline on the arterial wall.

Bypass surgery. If you have had traditional cardiac bypass surgery, you will be out of commission for a few weeks. You will probably arrive home wiped out and will gradually resume activity a bit at a time. The rate of your recovery will vary with many factors.

To start with, you must factor in your age, the presence of other diseases, and your individual tolerance for pain. There are also issues unique to surgery that you need to consider. Surgery is a major traumatic event to the body and it takes time for your tissues to heal. The healing period extends well beyond the time it takes for the anesthesia to wear off.

Also, most people who are placed on a heart-lung bypass machine will have some anemia, or reduction in red blood cells, after the procedure, which will increase feelings of fatigue. Anemia occurs because blood is lost in the heart bypass pump as well as during surgery itself. Blood transfusion is very effective for extreme cases of anemia, however the small but real risks associated with blood transfusion prevents its routine use for all patients after surgery. With proper nutrition or use of iron supplements, your blood level will return to normal within several weeks.

During your recovery, you will be encouraged to exercise more and more each day, and you may be referred to a formal program of cardiac rehabilitation. After angioplasty or bypass surgery, the cardiologist or surgeon who performed the procedure may want to see you for a follow up visit within several weeks to check for wound healing problems or other procedural complications.

Heart attack. If you have had a heart attack, with or without subsequent angioplasty or surgery, your doctor will put you on several new medications to improve your risk from further cardiac events. These may include medications to prevent blood clots, lower your heart rate or blood pressure, and medication to reduce your cholesterol. You will also be instructed on other lifestyle changes that will also improve your outlook. In addition, you will be given tests to evaluate your exercise tolerance, to measure the pumping power of your heart, and to analyze your heart rhythm.

You will be encouraged to exercise as much as you are able. Your doctor may recommend that you participate in a formal cardiac rehabilitation program.

Taking Control of Your Recovery

A couple of days after my husband got home after his bypass, we took a short walk to a bridge near our house. It was the longest walk of my life. He was the most ashen color. I thought I'd have to call the paramedics to get him home.
Lynn K.

Coming home from the hospital can be filled with uncertainty. In the hospital, your recovery was managed by a group of professionals. Medication appeared on schedule. Your diet was controlled by the nutritionist. The nurse supervised your activities and encouraged your progress. But now you actually are home, without your doctor, your nurse, your nutritionist, and all the rest of the support staff. Although you probably had some discussion of what happens when you finally get home, that discussion may not have prepared you for the anxiety and confusion you now face. You are probably asking yourself:

* *What pills do I take and when do I take them?*
* *What activities are appropriate?*
* *Should I join a cardiac rehabilitation program?*
* *What should I eat?*
* *What shouldn't I eat?*
* *When can I go back to work?*
* *Why don't I feel like myself?*

Despite your anxiety, this is a critical time for organizing your medical care and getting on the right track.

Resuming Your Normal Activities

Be patient with yourself as you begin to resume your normal activities. In general, avoid any activities that may strain your breastbone or tire you out, and rest between activities. Try to get 8 to 10 hours of sleep every night, and plan several rest periods each day. You don't need to go to bed or take a nap, just sit and relax for a little while.

Bathing. You can start bathing as soon as your incision has healed. Wash your incision gently with soap and water, but do not scrub. Also, avoid bathing in very hot water. It may help to place a heavy chair with rubber tips in the shower.

Climbing stairs. Take your time climbing stairs, and sit down to rest if you feel tired, short of breath, or dizzy.

Driving. Do not drive a car for about 4 to 6 weeks after surgery. Your reaction time will be slower due to fatigue and medication. Also, avoid long rides in the car for several weeks; stop every 1 to 2 hours to walk around.

Household chores. For the first 4 to 6 weeks after your surgery, avoid doing any chores that may put stress on the breastbone or are very tiring, such as vacuuming, gardening, shoveling snow, moving furniture, and doing laundry.

Lifting. Do not lift more than 5 to 10 pounds for 4 to 6 weeks after surgery. Also, don't try to unscrew tight jar lids, open stuck windows, or open heavy doors, as all of these things can strain your breastbone.

Maybe you are fortunate enough to have a family physician, internist, or cardiologist who you like and trust, and who is ready to provide this support. If not, it is important to your recovery that you to find someone you can work with. In addition to general support, you will need periodic electrocardiograms, blood evaluations, and other diagnostic tests to maximize your recovery.

Common Problems

In the months following a heart attack or revascularization procedure you may notice some changes in your emotional health or sexual function that seem unrelated to the diagnosis. These are actually common side effects of the life-changing event you have been through. It is important to discuss these issues with your doctor to receive treatment if it is available or to relieve some of the anxiety and discomfort that these conditions can cause.

Depression. Some researchers estimate that nearly 40 percent of people who have suffered a heart attack or coronary event experience depression afterward. Symptoms include: sleeplessness; loss of appetite; difficulty concentrating; feelings of hopelessness; no interest in relationships and activities you used to enjoy; or thoughts of death or suicide. Although many people feel down from time to time, depression is a clinical condition that lingers for more than just a couple of weeks and significantly interferes with your day-to-day life.

For many people, this depression may be a temporary condition, one that is related to the overwhelming adjustment to the reality of a cardiac diagnosis. For others, the depression triggered by a heart attack or coronary episode is long lasting and requires therapy or medical intervention.

Fatigue. Tiredness can certainly be one consequence of depression or anxiety, but in other circumstances it can be caused by the skeletal muscle weakness that naturally develops after a prolonged period of bed rest. Some of this fatigue can be caused by anemia, which is common after coronary bypass surgery. Also, some medications prescribed for acute coronary events may cause fatigue at the outset. While you may be able to successfully adapt over time, your doctor may have to change the medication or dose if fatigue persists. Fatigue may also stem from reduced pumping power of the heart, lowered blood pressure, or an irregular cardiac rhythm.

Between my wife's health stuff and my health stuff, we're like 75-year-olds. As far as sex, the doctors tend to talk about what's right for the man, what they think the man needs. And they give you these awful cartoon books. It's just not like that. I didn't have any type of impotence, I just didn't feel like having sex. Everything hurts. It took me a year and a half after surgery just to swing a golf club.
Lou S.

You can't hold someone tight when they've got a big scar on their chest. And you can't be as sexual when those surgeries take place. At those moments when you need closeness, that contact will be cut off. That's a normal part of recovery. And when you can't have sex, it doesn't mean that the person doesn't love you or need you. In fact, they need you more than ever.
Denise S., wife of Lou S.

Sexual dysfunction. Many people experience a loss of interest in sex in the weeks or months following a heart attack or revascularization. This can be the result of depression, medication, or the exhaustion that is common during recovery. Sexual desire and function may return as your health returns.

If you have taken Viagra (sildenafil citrate) in the past as an aid to sexual function, you will want to discontinue using it until you've met with your cardiologist to discuss possible negative effects in light of your diagnosis. Adverse reactions have been reported between sildenafil and short- or long-acting nitrate drugs (such as nitroglycerin) so potential drug-to-drug interactions should be discussed with your doctor.

Potential Dangers

We were following Dean Ornish's very low-fat diet. My husband had never weighed that much and he was losing a lot of weight on it. He got so thin, 150 pounds, which is small for someone who is 6 feet tall. We were careful until one night he ate half a bag of chocolate covered raisins. I felt so guilty about that. That night, I woke up enough to hear him

*calling me for help. He was on the floor, sweating from every pore. I'd never
seen anyone sweat like that. The kids were terrified. I called 911 and they
said, "Is he breathing?" And so I checked and he was. He crawled to the
bed and he looked terrible.*
Denise S.

After you've had a heart attack, your greatest risk in the weeks
following your return home from the hospital is an episode of
angina or another heart attack. This is most likely to occur in the first
24 hours after the initial attack, and is more likely to occur after a
severe heart attack that has caused significant damage to the heart
muscle. When the extent of heart muscle damage after a heart attack
is large, cardiac arrhythmias are an additional risk.

After angioplasty, with or without stent placement, your
greatest risk is that the treated artery may again become blocked.
This can happen either rapidly because of a blood clot or more
slowly because muscular scar tissue forms around the stent at the
site of the angioplasty. Scar tissue can sometimes produce an
even worse obstruction than existed before the procedure. This
blockage could reduce the flow of blood to a level that could
cause a heart attack. Fortunately, if this happens, it should
produce symptoms that will alert you and your doctor to the
problem in time to fix it.

Other potential consequences of heart disease include left
ventricular dysfunction, heart failure, occlusions in peripheral
arteries, rhythm irregularities, low blood pressure or extremely
low heart rate. You don't have to be able to diagnose any of these
conditions yourself, but it will be important for you to stay
attuned to symptoms that could signal serious complications.

*We can't define what my angina is. A couple of times I would have a sore
throat and my ears would hurt. A couple of times I woke up like that,
and it would be gone in a couple of hours. Those were the same symptoms I had with my heart attack. It happened again a couple of weeks
after I came home from the hospital, but they checked me into the hospital and there was nothing.*
Margaret G.

When to Call Your Doctor

You'll want to call your doctor if you experience these symptoms:

* *Angina*
* *Dizziness or marked confusion*
* *Persistent fever*
* *Prolonged recovery time from ordinary activities or exercise*
* *Rapid or irregular pulse*
* *Shortness of breath while at rest*
* *Swelling or drainage at any incision site*

Sometimes you will have or seem to have one of these symptoms and may call your doctor or even go to the hospital only to discover that what you are experiencing is a normal part of your recovery and nothing to worry about. Don't be embarrassed or ashamed if this happens. You are learning a new set of physical sensations that go along with your diagnosis. And there is nothing like a heart attack or bypass surgery to get you to pay attention to symptoms that never would have bothered you before. It is better to be overly cautious during your first weeks of recovery than to be too optimistic, and ignore symptoms that could signal a serious condition.

> *You can have gas pains and it will feel similar. Sometimes I think these cardiologists need to go through a heart attack and see what it's like. I'd like to go to a cardiologist who has been through this.*
> *Lou S.*

> *I was at work, and I was having some pain. I thought it might be gastrointestinal—that or angina. I took some nitro, and it felt like a big, fat elephant sat on my chest. I had to leave the room.*
> *Mary T.*

> *I was out in the garden one day, and I thought a boulder had hit me in the chest. It was like someone had put his hand in my chest and was squeezing it.*
> *Steven S.*

Is It Angina or a Heart Attack?

The classic symptoms of angina or of a heart attack are chest pain, characterized as tightness, squeezing, heaviness, or burning in the center of the chest. This pain may radiate to the back, arms, neck, and shoulders, and even up to the jaw. Associated with cardiac pain may be anxiety, weakness, nausea, rapid or irregular heart rate, difficulty breathing, or heavy sweating, or any combination of these.

Angina is temporary. Angina occurs when your heart needs more oxygen than it is getting. For this reason, angina is usually brought on by exercise. The problem corrects itself when you rest and reduce the heart's demand for oxygen. Angina usually goes away in less than 15 minutes, and often lasts only a minute or two.

Heart attack pain persists. When the blood supply to the heart is reduced to the point where the heart's need for oxygen cannot be met even while you are at rest, the muscle cells in the heart can begin to die. It usually takes more than 15 to 20 minutes for this condition to develop. For this reason, heart attack pain is usually distinguished from angina because it persists for a prolonged time, generally more than 30 minutes.

Your symptoms are unique to you. Women tend to experience more fatigue and nausea and less pain. They are somewhat less likely to experience chest pain, and may instead feel pain in the jaw, head, arms, or even elbows. Patients with diabetes sometimes feel no cardiac pain at all. Elderly patients are more likely to experience dizziness, confusion, difficulty breathing, and rapid pulse when they have angina or a heart attack. Becoming familiar with your symptoms and how your body feels when angina strikes will give you a better idea of how to modify your activity level and when to call your doctor.

Working Together with Your Doctor

After my emergency angioplasty, my internist referred me to a cardiologist, but we didn't hit it off. During our first meeting, the phone kept ringing

in his office, and not just that, there was a voice coming over his intercom asking for this or that. So he kept getting interrupted. He just didn't seem to be focused on me. And he said that he would never have given me an angioplasty, because at the time, back in 1996, it was a little bit riskier. Well, right away he was criticizing the doctors who had probably saved my life. I left his office and called the doctors in Washington who had worked on me and got them to recommend someone else. Now I have a doctor I like.
Demetre S.

If you're going to have a long-term relationship with a doctor, you have to think about your compliance to their suggestions. If you're high strung, you need someone who is meticulous about every aspect of your condition. If you're laid back, like me, then you need someone who's there when you need him, but not constantly causing worry.
Mary T.

It is important to remember that you have a choice of doctors to treat you. Of course, in an emergency, you want the most talented and experienced person to deal with the immediate problems. This may be a specialist who is based in a hospital intensive care area, or a cardiologist who is expert at performing complex urgent procedures, or a surgeon who has lots of experience doing operations on the heart.

But the immediate situation is not the only thing: You also need long-term continuity of care. The doctors who are critical to the short-term management of a crisis are not always the right people to take care of you for the long run.

A key step in taking control of your heart health is finding a doctor with whom you can have a productive long-term relationship. This is someone you'll feel comfortable talking to about both your symptoms and your fears. You will need someone who will listen to you and treat you with respect. And you'll need someone whose recommendations you respect. This may not be easy in the modern world of managed care, with its emphasis on shorter and shorter patient visits. But finding this type of relationship is critical to your health. If you don't like your doctor, you are less likely to follow his or her suggestions. You'll also be less likely to schedule and keep follow-up appointments or to take your medications. All of these things will have a negative effect on your long-term health.

You may already have a doctor you like and trust. If your heart disease is stable, ask your primary care doctor or internist if he or she is comfortable managing the medical details of your problem. Ask whether it would be appropriate to see a cardiologist from time to time, and under what conditions. Your doctor may be able to provide recommendations for a cardiologist. Another way to find a doctor is to ask friends about doctors in your community. If you have had a procedure done by a cardiologist or a surgeon, ask whom they would recommend for your long-term care. Make a routine appointment to see your regular doctor or cardiologist while your problem is stable, because you can get to know each other better in a non-emergency situation. If you have just come home from the hospital, now is the time to start looking for a medical team you can trust.

Ask a Lot of Questions

I've got this pain in my sternum area, and a sickly feeling with a little pain that moves over to the left shoulder. It happens any time of day and sometimes wakes me up at night. I want to ask my doctor if I can let this go or will it develop into a heart attack. This condition keeps me in a cautious state.
Dennis L.

A good doctor will try to educate you about your disease. But doctors vary in their ability to explain complex medical issues, just as patients have varying abilities as listeners. As a patient, you have a right and a responsibility to ask questions about what you need to know. You will need to know about your symptoms and sensations, about the medications you may be taking, and about the risks and benefits of the procedures you may have to undergo. Several studies have shown that patients who are able to talk to a doctor or nurse about their symptoms in the first few months after a heart attack make fewer trips to the emergency room and spend less time in the hospital than those who don't.

Know Your Medications

It can be very confusing to keep track of the cocktail of medications that your doctor has probably prescribed for you. Before you go home, make sure you know:

* *The names of your medications (it may be helpful to note both generic and brand name to avoid confusion when you go to the pharmacy)*

* *What it does*

* *How much to take*

* *When and how to take it*

* *What the possible side effects of each medication are*

* *What to do if you forget and miss a pill*

After a cardiac event, you will need to spend time learning which symptoms are benign and which might signal a potential problem. If you've had surgery, you'll need to learn to distinguish between the natural pain and fatigue of recovery and the pain of angina. Using your regularly scheduled appointments to discuss your questions is the best way to gain confidence that your recovery is proceeding on course.

Your Role in Recovery

In a way I've been pretty lucky. I didn't have a serious heart attack to start with. And I've gotten good care. But I also take care of myself. I quit smoking, I exercise, I'm trying to lose weight, and I'm enjoying retirement. At this stage the name of the game is staying alive.
Demetre S.

For my implanted defibrillator, I'm supposed to go in every 6 months, so they can check it. I once let it go for a year and they said, "Don't you dare do that again."
Ivan B.

A cardiologist, even a very gifted one, can do only so much for you. Ultimately, your health depends on your cooperation and attitude. Successful patients are the ones who take an active role in their own recovery. This often means making healthier lifestyle choices even if these choices are difficult to stick to. It also means being honest about the way your body feels and taking recommended diagnostic tests at regular intervals even if you feel fine. The more you do for yourself, the more your doctor can do for you.

The Role of Spouse and Family

Bypass surgery is such an intense experience for couples. They put him on the gurney and let us say good-bye. When they took him away, I remember looking at the floor and saying, "God, please don't let him die." I still cry when I think about it. It was a seven-hour surgery. I sat in the waiting room by myself because everyone else had to go home. At one point they came in and said, "It's okay; he's on the bypass machine." I realized that meant his heart had stopped and he had a machine breathing and circulating blood for him. At that moment I was so scared. I thought, "This isn't natural."
Denise S.

The diagnosis of heart disease can signal a stressful and difficult time for any family. Although heart disease is usually a manageable condition, it is also life-threatening. It is important for family members and especially caregivers to educate themselves about the causes of heart disease. Knowledgeable family members can be an enormous resource for patients as they strive to take medications correctly or to make difficult but important lifestyle changes.

It is also important for family members and caregivers to take care of themselves. The recovery period after a cardiac event or surgery can be as exhausting and emotionally draining for families as it is for the patient. Caregivers who can reach out to their friends and neighbors, to a therapist, or to members of the clergy for support and guidance will be better able to help both the patient and themselves manage the stress of a chronic condition.

Some Questions to Ask

Your primary task in the weeks following your diagnosis or hospitalization is to find a cardiologist you can work with in your recovery. You'll want to get references from your primary care physician, from friends who have been through similar circumstances, or from the surgeon who operated on you in the hospital. When you see your doctor, you'll want to have a list of questions ready to get a handle on your condition and on what you can expect in the coming months. Some examples of these questions are:

* *What tests were administered to me in the hospital and what were the results?*

* *What medications have I been given? What do they do? How long will I be taking them?*

* *Has my heart suffered significant damage? If so, in which areas? What are the long-term implications of this damage?*

* *Which tests, medications and other interventions do you normally recommend for someone in my situation?*

* *What physical symptoms, including pain, fatigue, and sleeplessness, are appropriate for my condition and which ones signal a problem that needs immediate attention?*

Chapter 3

◆ ◆ ❖ ◆ ◆ ❖ ◆ ◆ ❖ ◆ ◆ ❖ ◆ ◆ ❖ ◆ ◆ ❖ ◆ ◆

The Miracle of Modern Recovery
Advances in Treating Heart Disease

Many people being diagnosed today with heart disease came of age in the 1960s, when very little was known about the causes of heart attacks or how to prevent them. In this chapter, you'll read about the thinking that was current all those years ago and then to look at how dramatically treatment has evolved in the intervening decades. Although bypass surgery and angioplasty may seem to be the star developments of the past 45 years, the most important research has studied the causes of heart disease.

Because of this research, people can change their lifestyle in ways that help prevent heart attacks. Cardiologists can enhance these lifestyle changes with specific medications that further protect the heart and circulatory system. However, 50 years ago, it was much different.

My father had a heart attack in 1966, when he was 59. When they sent him home from the hospital, they didn't tell him to change his diet or quit smoking or anything like that, and he smoked a lot. They had even let him smoke in his hospital room. The doctor told him that he couldn't

drink beer anymore, I remember that. My dad didn't like that because he liked a beer on the weekend. They told him he could have whiskey instead, which he didn't like at all. He seemed fine, and then about six months later he had another heart attack. My mother and I took him to the hospital. After he was treated, he complained of pain. He told me to take my mother downstairs to get a cup of coffee right away. I think he knew he was dying, even though he told us he was fine. When we got back to the room, he was dead. I remember asking the doctor how this could have happened. He was in the hospital. The doctor said, "What are you talking about? He should have died the first time."
Ellen B.

My father died of heart disease when he was 55 or 56, the same age I was when I had my heart attack. That's relatively young. He had congestive heart failure, caused originally when he was a kid. He had rheumatic fever and that stayed with him his whole life. My mother had heart problems, too. So did my uncle. Still, I was afraid of heart disease because there wasn't anything anyone could do for them at the end but give them morphine.
Demetre S.

The Way Things Were

Back in the 1960s, when nearly half of all adults smoked and few had ever heard of cholesterol, heart disease was an increasingly common killer. At that time, the word "coronary" was sometimes considered to be synonymous with death. A person who collapsed at home or in public from a massive heart attack often died where he fell. Although cardiopulmonary resuscitation had been developed in the late 1950s, by the mid 1960s only a few doctors and nurses were trained to administer it. The external defibrillator, a machine designed to shock the heart to restart it after cardiac arrest, had been invented in 1955, but these machines were still large and cumbersome. Ambulances didn't carry them. Even in the hospital, defibrillators were too large to quickly move to the bedside of a patient in need.

In those days, there was no such thing as bypass surgery, or balloon angioplasty. There were no medical tests to diagnose heart disease and few medicines to treat patients in crisis. In the absence of what we consider to be standard medical care for coronary events, doctors had few choices. A patient admitted to the hospital with acute angina, or chest pain, and a suspected coronary thrombosis, or heart attack, was treated primarily with painkillers and complete bed rest.

Back then, doctors dulled the ache with drugs such as morphine, then put the patient to bed for up to 6 weeks with strict orders to remain still so as not to strain the ailing heart while it healed. Doctors knew that patients who suffered from one heart attack were at high risk for a potentially fatal arrhythmia within the first few days. To prevent this, beginning in the 1960s, doctors often moved heart patients to a single ward, called a coronary care unit (CCU).

In the CCU, patients with symptoms or signs of a heart attack were monitored 24 hours a day. If the ECG showed a wildly erratic heartbeat, called fibrillation, or if the patient's heart stopped, an alarm sounded and technicians appeared to perform CPR or deliver an electric shock to restart the heart. If a patient's blood pressure dropped too low, signaling imminent circulatory shock, doctors administered drugs that constricted the patient's arteries to bring blood pressure back to normal. They also administered drugs to increase the force of the heart's contractions, even though there was a great risk that these drugs would themselves produce tachycardia (rapid heart rate), fibrillation, or cardiac arrest. Doctors had no other choice. In those days, the use of nitroglycerin in the acute phase of a heart attack was discouraged because it was known to dilate the arteries and reduce blood pressure, which was thought to increase the risk of circulatory shock and death.

During the patient's long hospital stay, nurses were instructed to keep patients comfortable and sedated, and to minimize anxiety-producing phone calls and visitors. Patients were usually fed a lukewarm liquid diet during their hospitalization, as heavy meals and foods of extreme temperatures were thought to shock the heart.

In 1966, a classic textbook for treating heart patients was *Diseases of the Heart* by Charles K. Friedberg. In it, Friedberg outlines the reasoning behind this reactive style of medicine and extended hospitalization.

"The treatment of acute myocardial infarction is designed: (1) to reduce the work of the heart until the infarcted area is healed; (2) to alleviate pain or other discomfort; (3) to overcome shock and cardiac failure if present; and (4) to cope with dangerous cardiac arrhythmias or any complications that may arise."

This seems reasonable enough. But the scientific basis behind this treatment was as limited as the resources available to achieve these goals. After removing pain and its associated anxiety and enforcing bed rest, doctors turned to the task of preserving the oxygen-starved cells in the heart. This is not easy to do when there is no way to remove blockages from the coronary arteries. One experimental technique attempted to force oxygen into the system. For this, patients were sometimes put in an oxygen tent, filled with 95 percent to 100 percent oxygen at two to three atmospheres for a couple of hours at a stretch. This was not widely used, and it was known that exposure to high pressure oxygen for more than a couple of hours was toxic.

Blood Thinning Drugs Were Controversial

The role of blood clots in causing acute heart attacks was surprisingly controversial at the time. Although early studies indicated that many heart attacks were triggered by blood clots in one or more of the major coronary arteries, other studies suggested that blood clots might actually be the result, rather than the cause, of heart attacks.

Anticoagulant drugs were available at the time, but their use in the treatment of heart attacks in the mid-1960s varied widely. Doctors couldn't agree on which patients should receive them, or how much of these drugs to use. Many doctors rightly worried that anticoagulants would cause internal bleeding in some patients.

In addition, many doctors disliked the so-called rebound effect of anticoagulants. Although these drugs would prevent blood clots in the short term, doctors knew that as soon as the drug was discontinued, the patient would temporarily be at increased risk for developing a life-threatening blood clot. In light of this, many doctors felt that the immediate survival benefit was not worth this risk.

Friedberg, by contrast, was highly in favor of using anticoagulants, saying that anything that improved survival rates was an important tool of treatment. He prescribed them to all of his patients unless he felt that they were at particular risk for suffering internal bleeding. He even used them to treat patients showing signs of an imminent heart attack, feeling that these drugs would prevent blood clots that were still forming. For some patients he prescribed long-term anticoagulant therapy, a concept that was ahead of its time.

Complications Were Difficult to Treat

Treating the other complications resulting from heart attacks was more problematic in Friedberg's day. The two main complications of a heart attack (assuming that the patient survived long enough to be admitted to the hospital) were irregular heart rhythms, called arrhythmias, and heart failure. Heart failure occurs when the heart muscle suffers such extensive damage that it is unable to pump adequately.

Arrhythmias can be separated into two groups: Those that cause death by making the heart beat too rapidly, such as ventricular tachycardia and ventricular fibrillation; and others, such as heart block, that caused death by making the heart beat too slowly.

At the end of the 1960s, doctors in coronary care units used several drugs to suppress abnormal rhythms that could lead to death. These drugs were most effective in treating arrhythmias that led to abnormally fast heart rates. Arrhythmias that caused slow heart rates did not respond to defibrillators or drug treatment alone. Methods to stimulate the slowed heart were pretty primitive and clumsy. Permanently implantable pacemakers were still relatively new and not widely used.

There was little that doctors could do to treat severe heart failure or shock associated with heart attacks, and nothing they could do to remove blockages of the arteries themselves. Attempting surgery on a beating heart was still a radical concept in the mid-1960s, something researchers were busy perfecting in laboratories—on dogs. Surgeons did remove blood clots from the arteries of the arms and legs, because a complete arterial blockage in this area could be serious enough to cause the affected limb to die. Still, limbs could be held still for surgery, and surgeons had not developed a method for working directly on the heart. During and after a heart attack, the blockages in coronary arteries stayed where they were.

Recovery Was an Alien Concept

Through the 1960s, when patients finally were sent home, after weeks or sometimes months in the hospital, they were told to "take it easy." That meant resting several times a day and avoiding any activities that would labor the heart, including housework, yard work, walking, and sex. Many patients were urged to retire from work and discouraged from exercising or returning to athletic activities they once enjoyed. Although doctors knew that weeks of bed rest followed by months or years of restricted activity caused anxiety and depression in most patients, they believed that any other course could bring on another, perhaps fatal, heart attack.

While patients may have been told to lose some weight or to cut down on their cigarette smoking, fatty foods, or salt intake, they were often given no real guidelines about how or why to do that. Although researchers in the now-famous Framingham Heart Study had already discovered astonishing correlations between heart disease and such factors as high blood pressure, high total cholesterol, obesity, diabetes, stress, and genetics, it was not clear that those risk factors could be modified, or that doing so would improve the natural history of coronary artery disease. It was also unknown how much effect lifestyle modifications, such as diet and exercise, would have on established heart disease.

Studies on the health factors associated with heart disease had already confirmed that smokers were at much higher risk for heart attacks and sudden coronary death as early as 1960. In 1964, the surgeon general had even issued a warning label for cigarette packages, telling smokers that they were at risk for heart disease and lung cancer. Soon, the tobacco industry was busy selling the idea that filters would offer some protection from these health hazards.

Not surprisingly, given the advice they received, many patients who survived their hospital stay went home and died of subsequent heart attacks or strokes as their heart disease progressed unchecked. There was nothing else that could be done. Doctors told their patients that they were lucky to be alive and that they should go home and enjoy whatever life they could carve out for themselves, no matter how unsatisfactory or unrecognizable that life was.

> *After I had my bypass surgery, I went to a club and sat at a table with four men I have known for many years. All journalists. They said, "Where have you been?" I opened my shirt and showed them my scar, at which point, they all opened their shirts and showed me identical scars. It made me feel very much at home.*
> *Dennis L.*

Forty Years of Amazing Progress

Now, decades later, a person who survives a heart attack or who is diagnosed with heart disease really is lucky to be alive at a time when so much is known about the circulatory system and how to protect it from further damage. Today, the major goal of therapy when a person enters the hospital with a heart attack is to restore blood flow to the heart muscle through the obstructed coronary artery as quickly and as completely as is possible. Early restoration of blood flow can limit or prevent the major complications of a heart attack and will reduce the amount of damage done to the heart muscle itself.

Bypassing Blockages with Surgery

The modern era of heart disease diagnosis and surgery was already emerging when Friedberg wrote the final edition of his book in 1966. The very next year, Soviet surgeons completed the first coronary artery bypass operation on a beating heart, and the first report of the procedure using heart-lung bypass by Rene Favaloro appeared in an American medical journal in 1969. The heart-lung bypass is a machine that performs all the functions of the heart and lungs, keeping oxygenated blood moving through the body while the heart is temporarily stopped.

In the classic coronary artery bypass operation, surgeons open the chest, stop the heart, and work directly on the coronary arteries to reroute blood around the blockages. In this way, doctors can restore blood flow to the parts of the heart threatened by blockages of plaque or blood clots. Surgeons had much greater success working on those tiny coronary arteries when the heart itself would sit still. Currently, surgeons complete about 400,000 bypass surgeries each year, now often using arteries in addition to, or in place of, veins alone. Long-term studies indicate that arteries tend to last longer than veins as bypass vessels.

As surgical techniques have improved, surgeons have even begun to circumvent the bypass machine and some are now performing bypass surgery without using the heart-lung machine. This surgery, called off-pump coronary bypass, is once again performed on the beating heart. Avoiding the bypass machine has several benefits. Not only do patients generally have a smaller scar, but the surgery itself is less of an ordeal. The heart doesn't have to be stopped at the beginning of surgery and then restarted again at the end. Also, the circulation to the organs is provided by the heart, rather than by an artificial pump, so many of the side effects associated with the heart lung machine might be avoided, including post-operative confusion, anemia, and bleeding. On the other hand, these limited incision, off bypass operations sometimes do not provide the exposure and control that a surgeon may need to do complete revascularization of the heart. Only the lowest risk patients may be candidates for this surgery.

Looking Inside the Arteries

In the late 1960s, doctors began to experiment with a new technique for measuring pressures in the chambers of the heart and taking x-ray pictures of the insides of the chambers and the main arteries of the body, including the coronary arteries, called cardiac catheterization. This technique originated in the 1930s when a young German doctor, named Werner Forssmann inserted a thin rubber tube into his own arm and advanced it upward into his heart. He documented his achievement when he walked into the x-ray department and took a picture of the catheter in place. Since that time, catheters in the heart have become an indispensable part of cardiac medicine. They can be used to measure pressures in the atria and ventricles and in the large arteries, or to inject substances directly into different parts of the circulatory system. A specialized form of catheterization involves angiography, in which x-ray pictures are taken after the injection of a dye that outlines the walls of blood vessels. During the 1960s it became possible to perform selective angiography of the coronary arteries. This coronary angiography allowed obstructions of the vessels to be visualized, creating a "road map" for defining and ultimately treating coronary artery disease. At least 1.3 million diagnostic catheterization procedures are performed each year in the United States. Many of these are now conducted on an outpatient basis.

In 1977, a physician in Switzerland discovered a way to use this catheterization to remove blockages. Andreas Gruenzig put a small balloon on the end of a catheter and threaded it into a coronary artery. When the balloon was inflated, it opened the blockage and restored blood flow through the artery. The procedure became known as percutaneous transluminal coronary angioplasty (PTCA), and at least 500,000 now are performed every year. This number is growing rapidly.

Opening Blocked Arteries

In 1986 a surgeon in France created another innovation in treatment using a modified dental prosthesis. Jacques Puel placed a metallic cylinder, called a stent, into a coronary artery to hold it open and restore blood flow. Currently, more than 70 percent of angioplasty procedures include stenting to open blocked arteries. In fact, more than 400,000 stents were implanted in the year 2000. In the early years of angioplasty and stenting the major problem was that the arteries treated suffered a 20 to 30 percent rate of "restenosis," the subsequent return of blockage in the artery. The problem of restenosis has been dramatically reduced by newer stents, called drug eluting stents. These stents contain drugs that are slowly released into the artery to prevent smooth muscle cells and scar tissue from building up at the site of the stent and ultimately blocking the artery again.

During these decades cardiac pacemakers were improving as well—becoming lighter and more effective. In 1985, the FDA approved a new device, called the implantable cardioverter-defibrillator (ICD) that was designed to monitor each heartbeat, like a regular pacemaker. But unlike regular pacemakers, ICDs are capable of terminating ventricular tachycardia and ventricular fibrillation by delivering a shock to the heart to restore a normal heart rhythm, for people at high risk for ventricular fibrillation, while the biventricular pacemaker uses synchronized pacing of the heart to better stimulate the heart's normal electrical activity.

Advances in the ER

In addition to these tools for treating the complications from heart disease, researchers have also developed better ways to treat people who come to the emergency room with a suspected heart attack. These include:

* *Lab tests to confirm or rule out a heart attack.*
* *Clot-busting drugs and antiplatelet medications to remove existing clots and prevent future clots.*
* *Medications that control heart rate and blood pressure to preserve heart muscle cells and reduce the likelihood of another heart attack.*
* *Non-invasive procedures such as a thallium scan, echocardiogram, and ultrasound to find and assess arterial blockages or heart function.*

Treatment for heart disease has also moved outside the hospital and into the public places where many heart attacks occur. Today, a person who suffers a sudden heart attack in a public place such as a mall or health club or even a restaurant may receive life-saving CPR from a trained bystander.

Emergency medical technicians called to a scene of a suspected MI are ready to use a defibrillator to shock the heart into pumping again if it has stopped. There are also automatic defibrillators in many public places, including casinos, health clubs, police cars, commercial aircraft, and in most airport terminals. These can be used by personnel who are not specifically medically trained.

> *I was in my office, at my desk. I was on the phone and got some chest pain. I was talking to my wife who was in the hospital visiting her mother. My wife put her mother's doctor on the phone and he talked to me for a couple of minutes. Finally, he said, "Get to the hospital right now. I'll have somebody waiting for you there." Of course, it was noon and I couldn't get a cab. I finally hailed a limo and the driver got stuck in traffic. He dropped me off at the wrong corner. All this time, 30 minutes or so, the pain was getting worse. Walking to the hospital entrance, I had to stop a couple of times and lean on to the building to rest. When I got into the emergency room, the doctor who walked up to meet me was a cardiologist. He said, "You're in good hands," and that's all I remember before I passed out.*
> Ivan B.

Recovery Is Faster

In 1966, a patient hospitalized for myocardial infarction spent up to six weeks in the hospital. Today, a patient who has a heart attack but no subsequent complications such as arrhythmia or ongoing angina might be in the hospital for just a few days. Two decades ago, a patient undergoing bypass surgery might spend two weeks in the hospital. Now, a patient undergoing elective bypass surgery is likely to be sent home from the hospital after just five days, while a patient undergoing angioplasty to receive a stent might be home the following afternoon. Under a doctor's supervision, each of these individuals can resume many of his or her ordinary activities—including driving and working—within a month. In the case of a simple angioplasty or stent procedure where there is no heart attack, the patient might be back at work in a day or two.

Survival Has Improved Dramatically

These medical advances have contributed to a dramatic reduction in the number of deaths resulting from heart disease. The rate of coronary heart disease deaths in Americans has decreased by 56 percent since 1950. If the rate of coronary heart disease fatalities had remained at its 1963 level, an additional 621,000 people would die of heart disease each year. But those numbers may be conservative. The Minnesota Heart Survey found that the rate of mortality decreased 70 percent between 1970 and 1997, and that it decreased 50 percent between 1985 and 1997 alone. In addition, the study also showed that people are living much longer after they return home from the hospital.

It's tempting to think that people are faring better after heart attacks because of better hospital care and surgical techniques, such as bypass surgery and stenting. This is not the whole story. Indeed, much of the improvement in survival over recent decades is due to advances in the prevention of heart disease. These developments include new medications for treating disease and lifestyle changes that dramatically slow the progression of heart disease.

Chapter 4

◆ ◆ ❖ ◆ ◆ ❖ ◆ ◆ ❖ ◆ ◆ ❖ ◆ ◆ ❖ ◆ ◆ ❖ ◆ ◆

What Is Heart Disease?
An Overview of the Current Understanding of Atherosclerosis

Atherosclerosis? Unstable angina? Endothelial cell function? Ejection fraction? A diagnosis of heart disease means facing a whole new vocabulary for your condition, and a simple tour of the circulatory system may help.

In this chapter you'll learn what the arteries do, why arterial plaque forms, how it blocks arteries, and—more important—how even minor blockages can make your arteries less efficient at moving blood. You'll learn about the causes of angina, the specific triggers for heart attacks, and the long-term consequences of untreated heart disease.

All of this information will help you to ask more specific questions of your doctor, and to better understand the results of any tests you take. You will also gain a clearer understanding of how the medications and interventions in Parts II and III work to prevent heart attacks and to slow the progression of heart disease.

The Heart at Work

The heart is a pump. Actually, it's two connected muscular pumps working side by side. The right side pumps blood to the lungs where

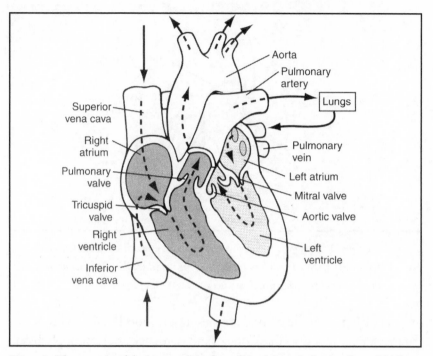

Figure 1: The structure of the heart and the flow of blood through the chambers of the heart. The left ventricle receives oxygenated blood from the lungs across the mitral valve from the left atrium and pumps it across the aortic valve into the major arteries.

it can pick up oxygen and get rid of carbon dioxide. The left side pumps this oxygen-rich blood through arteries to all the organs of the body (see Figure 1). The de-oxygenated blood returns from the body's organs through veins to the right side of the heart. Both sides rely on the same electrical stimulus—the body's natural pacemaker—to trigger the heart muscle to contract and push the blood along. After each contraction the heart muscle relaxes and receives the blood that will be ejected by the next contraction. At a heart rate of 60 to 90 beats per minute, the normal heart contracts about 100,000 times each day. That's a lot of work, and it takes a lot of energy for the heart to circulate the blood at rest and during exercise.

When oxygen-rich blood leaves the left ventricle of the heart, it flows through the aorta (the main artery leading from the left ventricle) to large arteries that serve as the major pathways of the circulatory system. These arteries are named for the part of the body

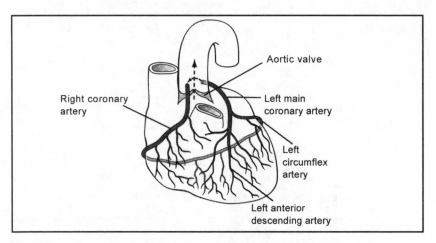

Figure 2: A schematic view of the major coronary arteries, which originate from the aorta. The left main coronary artery divides into two main branches: the left anterior descending artery to the front and the left circumflex artery to the back of the heart.

they serve. For example, carotid arteries supply blood to the brain. Renal arteries supply blood to the kidneys, and coronary arteries supply blood to the heart muscle. Major arteries divide into smaller arteries, which divide into yet smaller arterioles, and finally, into the tiny capillaries that feed blood directly to tissues and organs. From the capillaries in the organs of the body, the blood flows to small veins, then into increasingly larger veins until it reaches the right side of the heart. The blood then goes through the lungs once again, to begin the cycle again.

The Heart's Oxygen Supply

Even though the heart is full of blood, it gets its own oxygen-containing blood supply from special arteries that branch off the aorta, just like other muscles of the body. There are two coronary artery trunks that stem from the root of the aorta. (See Figure 2.) One of these is the right coronary artery, which supplies blood to the right ventricle and to several sections of the left ventricle. The other is the left main coronary artery, which divides into two additional major coronary artery branches. The left anterior descending coronary artery provides blood to the front and the sides of the left ventricle, as well as the wall of muscle tissue that divides the two ventricles. This dividing wall, called the septum, normally squeezes in coordination with the left ventricle. The other branch, called the left circumflex artery, provides blood to the rest of the left ventricle. These areas of supply overlap partially, so that some areas of the heart can be supplied by more than one artery.

How the Body's Oxygen Demand Is Met

At rest, the heart only needs to pump enough oxygen containing blood to the body to support the basic energy requirements of the muscles and other organs. With exercise, the oxygen requirement of the muscles of the body may increase many times, to 12 to 14 times the resting level. How do the muscles and the heart adapt to this increase in demand for oxygen in the circulating blood?

The normal heart can increase its output by increasing both the amount of blood ejected with each contraction and the number of contractions each minute. First, muscular exercise causes your blood to move faster in your system, particularly in the veins, where the blood is normally moving fairly slowly. Exercise also increases the force of each of your heartbeats and decreases the resistance to blood flow in the arteries. Together these factors cause the volume of blood ejected by the normal heart, its "stroke volume," to increase to about one and a half times the resting amount. Second, the harder you exercise, the faster your heart will beat (up to a point). In relatively young people, the heart rate during extreme exercise may increase from a resting rate of 60 beats per minute to about 180 beats per minute. So changing heart rate alone can increase the output of the heart by about three times the normal amount. Together, increases in stroke volume and heart rate during exercise can boost the output of the heart by about four and a half fold.

But the body's need for oxygen during peak exercise increases 12- to 14-fold, not four and a half-fold. Where does the rest of the oxygen supply to the body's major muscles come from? The answer is that the working muscles themselves can increase the amount of oxygen they extract from the blood by about three-fold. At rest, the muscles may extract only about a quarter of the oxygen present in arterial blood, but during the demand of exercise, this extraction can reach three-quarters. This increase in oxygen extraction can have profound consequences for patients with heart disease. Even if your heart is too damaged or weakened to increase its ability to pump blood, your muscles can make up the difference by increasing the amount of oxygen they take from the blood.

Calculating Your Heart Rate

Your resting heart rate is the number of times your heart beats in one minute when you are at complete rest. The best time to get an accurate resting heart rate is usually right after you wake up, before you even get out of bed. Using your pointer and/or middle fingers, count the beats in your pulse for 15 seconds and multiply by four. Or, you can use a heart rate monitor. Take these measurements for five consecutive days and find the average. This is your resting heart rate. Your resting heart rate varies depending upon your exercise routines, eating habits, quality of sleep, stress levels, and other factors. The fitter you are, the less effort and fewer beats per minute your heart requires to pump blood throughout your body.

Your maximum heart rate is the highest number of times your heart can beat in one minute. Maximum heart rate decreases with age, and is also reduced by beta-blocking drugs. The most accurate way of determining your maximum heart rate is to have your cardiologist administer a treadmill stress test. But you can also use the following "age-adjusted formula" to predict your maximum heart rate.

Maximum HR= 220 minus your age (in years)

For example, if you are a 55-year-old man, your age-adjusted maximum heart rate is 220 minus 55 years = 165 bpm (beats per minute).

This formula is usually accurate to within 10 to 15 beats per minute. Like your resting heart rate, your maximum heart rate is affected by a variety of factors, including heredity and fitness level.

The Heart's Unique Needs

Just as the skeletal muscles require more oxygen to do more exercise, so the heart muscle requires more oxygen-rich blood to be able to pump harder and faster during exercise.

The difference is that skeletal muscles at rest use only a small fraction of the oxygen delivered by their arteries. During exercise, these muscles can simply use more of the oxygen they receive (up to three times as much) without needing more blood flow. Unlike skeletal muscle, however, the heart is moving all the time. It extracts and uses most of the oxygen from its arteries even when you are not exercising. This means that when your body demands more work and more output by your heart, that increased demand must be matched by an increase in flow through the coronary arteries.

When the coronary arteries are healthy, exercise causes them to dilate so that more blood gets to the heart muscle. But when coronary arteries cannot dilate, or when something inside the artery partially blocks blood flow, exercise becomes a problem: The increased energy demand of the heart may not be matched by an adequately increased blood supply through the coronary arteries. Indeed, it is not just exercise that can provoke this imbalance, but emotional stress as well, and other factors that increase the work of the heart, such as high blood pressure, can further compound this imbalance.

If you have heart disease, the blood supply to your heart is probably limited by atherosclerosis, a condition that blocks the coronary arteries and may make them less able to dilate during exercise. This leads to angina, unstable angina, and heart attacks.

What Is Atherosclerosis?

Often called arterial plaque, or hardening of the arteries, atherosclerosis is the gradual build-up of fat and fibrous material within the inner lining of the arteries. The condition progressively obstructs, or blocks, arterial vessels. Atherosclerosis affects the large and medium sized arteries of the body, including the aorta, the coronary arteries, the carotid arteries, the renal arteries, and the arteries that supply blood to the legs and feet. Arterial plaque isn't distributed evenly along the walls of arteries. Rather, it builds the way silt does in a stream, more in some areas and less in others, so that you might have a 90-percent blockage in one small section of an artery, while much of the rest of the artery may only show a 15-percent obstruction.

The build-up of plaque used to be thought of as a natural byproduct of aging. Now doctors know that it is a chronic disease that involves complex interactions between the arterial wall and various substances in the blood that produce an inflammatory-like response to injury. What causes arterial plaque to form? There are several theories, each of which is based on an exaggerated response of the body to real or perceived injury, toxins in the blood, or infection.

First Theory: Arterial Injury

One theory suggests that the arteries naturally sustain injuries from high blood pressure or toxins such as cigarette smoke.

Your body has a highly efficient system for repairing any type of tissue damage. The process is similar to what happens with a cut on your skin. Any rip or tear inside an artery attracts blood platelets (a type of blood cell that initiates blood clotting) and macrophages (a type of white blood cell that responds to toxins or infection) to the area. Blood platelets are programmed to initiate healing by sticking together on an injured surface. They do this whenever they locate a potential internal injury. By doing so, they create the first important step toward forming a blood clot that will stop internal bleeding.

Macrophages have a more complex role, that of fighting infection. They are attracted to the site of injury or tissue disturbance, where they enter the wall of the artery and consume foreign substances or toxins. Inside the vessel wall, they may consume LDL cholesterol particles and other toxins, which causes them to become larger "foam cells." In response, the lining of the arterial walls swell with irritation. In all of this activity, the macrophages, along with free-floating cholesterol particles, calcium particles and any other debris traveling in the blood stream, can get absorbed or trapped within and along the arterial wall. This mix of substances becomes arterial plaque. (See Figures 3 and 4.)

Second Theory: Low-Density Lipoprotein Particles

This theory suggests that the primary culprit in this cycle of plaque formation is the low-density lipoprotein particles (LDL or "bad"

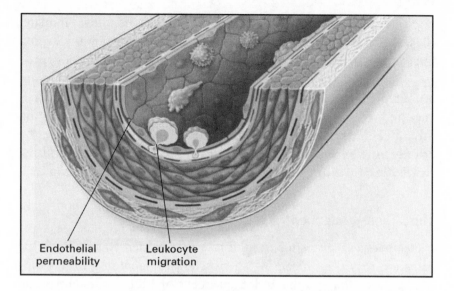

Endothelial
permeability

Leukocyte
migration

Figure 3: Early arterial abnormalities in atherosclerosis. These include permeability of the inner arterial wall (the endothelium) to white blood cells (leukocytes) and lipids.

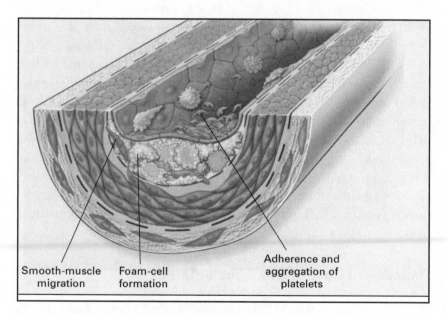

Smooth-muscle
migration

Foam-cell
formation

Adherence and
aggregation of
platelets

Figure 4: Development of an atherosclerotic plaque, with foam cell formation in the inner arterial wall compounded by the attraction and adherence of platelets and invasion by smooth muscle cells from deeper in the arterial wall.

cholesterol) circulating in the blood stream. As they circulate, these particles may enter the arterial wall, where they undergo a chemical reaction called oxidation. Oxidized LDL are devoured by scavenger-type blood cells called macrophages, which are attracted to the inner lining of the artery by the abnormal fat. Ingested oxidized LDL converts these macrophage cells to bulging "foam cells" that swell within the arterial wall. In this theory, the arteries narrow because they are chronically irritated by an inflammatory response to excess cholesterol in its oxidized LDL form.

Third Theory: Infection

Researchers are also studying the role that hidden bacterial or viral infection may play in causing atherosclerosis. According to this theory, it's not injury to the endothelial cells or LDL cholesterol alone that initiates the buildup of plaque. Rather, chronic infections cause the initial damage to the arterial wall that leads to the atherosclerotic accumulation of fat and debris. It is a controversial, but attractive, idea. It is supported—but not proved—by elevated levels of C-reactive protein (CRP) in patients with atherosclerosis. CRP is a marker for inflammation and infection. A few studies have tried to link coronary disease with gingivitis, a chronic infection of the gums. Other infections that have generated suspicious interest include C pneumoniae, a cause of pneumonia, cytomegalovirus, helicobacter pylori, a cause of stomach ulcer, and herpes simplex virus. Other researchers believe that it is the process of inflammation, rather than the specific infection, that is implicated by these studies. Of course, all three of these theories may be true, meaning that plaque may be caused primarily by injury, by excess cholesterol, or by inflammation, or perhaps to a combination of factors.

Decades of Destructive Accumulation

In most people, arterial plaque builds over many years. Some deposits have more cholesterol particles, or fatty streaks, while others have more hardened elements of plaque, called fibrous tissue. Over time, some deposits may solidify, or harden, and therefore

Antioxidants Against LDL

Oxidation is a normal chemical process in the cells of the body. Unfortunately, the oxidation of LDL particles results in a toxic irritant for the arteries and fosters the production of abnormal foam cells in the artery wall that can lead to arterial plaques. It is therefore logical to think that chemicals that reduce abnormal oxidation, known as "antioxidants," might block this process in the arterial wall.

A number of vitamins and other substances can act as antioxidants. In experimental studies of arterial cells, antioxidants have reduced the production of oxidized LDL and limited the development of early atherosclerosis. However, there is often a difference between experimental findings in test tubes and actual results in humans. For example, there was once considerable excitement about vitamin E as an antioxidant that might prevent the development of atherosclerosis, and for a number of years it was widely recommended for heart patients. As it turns out, most of the clinical data has shown that it does not have much beneficial effect on the cardiac event rate in people. It is possible that the doses used in these studies were not adequate, but they should have been.

One antioxidant that is attracting a lot of attention these days is vitamin (or co-enzyme) Q-10 (ubiquinone). In addition to antioxidant properties, Q-10 can increase the levels of high energy substances in heart muscle. An additional reason for attention to Q-10 replacement is that some of the lipid-lowering drugs, known as statins, seem to reduce the levels of Q-10 in the body. Therefore, some researchers theorize that people who have atherosclerosis, and particularly those who take statins, may benefit from taking Q-10 supplements. However, at the present time, there is no convincing evidence that Q-10 supplementation actually affects clinical events, but this is being actively studied and should be watched for outcome data.

A similar lack of convincing data exists for vitamin C.

Other substances, called flavanoids, have antioxidant properties. Flavanoids are found in wine, separate from alcohol, and in grape juice. This might explain the beneficial effects reported from moderate wine and juice intake, but further cause and effect studies are needed here. Flavanoids are also present in fruits, nuts, and vegetables. Another class of antioxidants, known as carotenoids, is found in carrots and in other yellow, red, and green fruits and vegetables. These are sensible to eat, but there are no data on their direct effects on coronary disease.

reduce the elasticity the arteries need to help move the blood.

Most arterial plaques do not obstruct much of the blood vessel in which they occur, although with enough time some can become large enough to interfere with blood flow in the artery. These plaques are sometimes called "stable," because they are less likely to rupture or tear. Those atherosclerotic deposits comprised mainly of fatty streaks are often called "unstable" because they are more prone to rupture, causing them to release their contents into the blood stream and trigger a blood clotting response that may completely obstruct the artery.

A plaque rupture in one of the coronary arteries that supplies blood to the muscle of the heart is usually the initial event in a heart attack, which then leads to a localized clot that completely blocks the blood flow to part of the heart muscle.

A Disease with Symptom-Free Beginnings

My brother ran four miles a day. He climbed mountains, didn't smoke or drink. He had low cholesterol and no symptoms of heart disease, no angina, and then he died one day of a massive heart attack. It was so shocking. He was only 53. At the autopsy, they found 90 percent blockage in one artery and an 80 percent blockage in another artery. I thought it might be genetic, because my father also died of heart disease when he was 67. I went to my doctor and took a stress test and it didn't show anything significant, I graded out at the 90th percentile, but my doctor sent me to a cardiologist anyway, because of my history. The cardiologist gave me a nuclear stress test. It indicated some blockage in one artery, so I had an angioplasty with a stent. I consider my brother unlucky. If he'd had symptoms or any of the risk factors, he would have gone to the doctor. Oscar M.

I was a runner for 20 years. I ran the boardwalk in Brooklyn every day. I ran the marathon in October 1981, three months before my daughter got married. In January of 1982 I was in the hospital recovering from a heart attack. I was 51 years old. At the time, even the doctors didn't know why I'd had a heart attack. Since then, I've had a bypass, an implantable defibrillator, and an angioplasty. This heart of mine is still working. Ivan B.

I had no previous history of heart disease. My blood pressure was high, which I knew. I did have what they call airport angina. I traveled the world for 40 years. As you get older, as you're walking down these concourses, every once in a while I had to set down my suitcase and look at the window displays, because I was a little out of breath. Doctors joke about that, and it was happening to me.
Tim S.

One of the problems with diagnosing and treating atherosclerosis is that it generally builds so slowly that many people do not notice any symptoms until the moment they suffer a first cardiovascular event. A first event could be the development of chest pain with exercise, called angina, if the oxygen demanded by the working heart muscle exceeds the supply that reaches the heart through the partially blocked coronary artery. Alternatively, a first event might be a heart attack if the unstable plaque leads to plaque rupture and clot that results in blockage of a coronary artery. Or, a stroke may occur if the main problem arises in the arteries leading to the brain.

Few, if any, of these young soldiers in the study mentioned below would have suspected that they were developing heart disease. Most people who have significant deposits of arterial plaque have no idea that something is wrong. As the disease progresses, and the arteries become

---

What the Research Shows

In 1953, during the war in Korea, U.S. Army researchers conducted what is now a classic study of the origins of atherosclerosis. They autopsied 300 young soldiers killed in action and carefully examined their coronary arteries. Although these soldiers had an average age of 22 and presumably no symptoms of heart disease, 77 percent of them already had visible evidence of atherosclerosis in their coronary arteries. Most of this evidence consisted of simple fatty streaks on the lining of arteries, without obstructive plaque. But of the 300 men autopsied, 9 percent had plaque deposits that narrowed a coronary artery by more than 50 percent, and 3 percent of them had complete blockages in one of the coronary arteries.

narrower and more calcified, some people do experience symptoms. For instance, exercise-related cramps in the legs may indicate that arterial plaque is decreasing blood supply to the major muscles of your legs. This is called peripheral arterial disease. Chest pain associated with effort or stress, called angina, may be a sign of coronary artery obstruction by arterial plaque. It is important to remember, though, that it is possible to have significant blockage in several coronary or peripheral arteries, or even a complete blockage in an artery, and suffer no pain or symptoms of any kind.

> *Strangely enough, I did have some chest pain about four weeks before my heart attack. It was a cold, windy afternoon. I was going to see a client, and I turned a corner and got a sharp pain in my chest. I thought I'd better go check it out. I went to my wife's mother's doctor. He gave me an ECG and told me that I was having angina, and sent me home. Less than four weeks later I had the heart attack.*
> Ivan B.

What Causes Angina?

At first, atherosclerosis appears as simple fatty streaks that line the arteries. These generally have no impact on coronary blood flow. Even when plaque blocks half the diameter of the coronary artery, more than enough blood generally gets through to supply the need of the heart muscle for energy during most daily activities, including moderate exercise. There is certainly enough blood to supply the heart at rest. In this situation, most people experience no symptoms.

But over time, layers of plaque continue to build. When the obstruction blocks 50 to 75 percent of the cross-sectional area of the artery, the blood supply to the heart muscle may still be more than adequate for the heart muscle at rest.

Still, the heart needs to increase its oxygen supply several times a day during exercise or in times of stress. When the escalator is broken and you need to walk up a flight of stairs, when you are carrying groceries in from the car, when you go out for a jog or a game of tennis, or when you get into a heated argument, your heart needs more oxygen. In these times, the narrowed arteries won't allow any more blood to get to those heart cells. When the heart needs more oxygen from the blood than it is getting, its cells literally ache for oxygen, and the resulting pain is called angina. If this occurs primarily during periods of strenuous exercise and extreme stress, it is called effort angina. This condition usually signals a moderate blockage in one or more of the major coronary arteries.

> *Now I have this angina, which has no sense to it. I can go down on a morning and play tennis, and take a nitro beforehand even if I don't need it. They tell me to take a tablet before exercise. I can go all day and have no problem at all, and then sit down and on getting up, and it strikes a note somewhere. Or I can be asleep and it will awaken me. And it disturbs me.*
> *Dennis L.*

Although angina can be extremely painful, even debilitating for some people, it rarely lasts for more than 10 minutes. When you stop exercising and rest, or when you calm down, your heart will need less oxygen to support the reduced level of activity and your circulatory system will eventually right the oxygen imbalance. A dose of nitroglycerin may help dilate the arteries to relieve your symptoms by increasing blood flow to the heart and decreasing the workload of the heart. However, if your body cannot correct this imbalance then some of the cells in the heart that have been starved of oxygen will become injured and may actually die. This is called a myocardial infarction—or a heart attack.

Atherosclerosis: The Traditional View

According to the traditional view of atherosclerosis, symptoms should increase in severity slowly and progressively over time as arterial obstruction builds gradually within the affected vessel. Angina should first occur during extreme exercise, when the heart's demand for oxygen is greatest. Over time, as arterial plaque continues to build greater obstructions within the artery, these symptoms would occur during more moderate exercise. Sooner or later progressive obstruction of the coronary artery should reduce blood supply to a level required just by the resting needs of the heart. If your angina occurs while you are at rest or awakens you from sleep, or seems totally unrelated to activity or emotional upset, it is called unstable angina. It signals near total blockage in one or more coronary arteries and it needs immediate medical attention.

The traditional theory of coronary artery disease predicts the slow build up of plaque that first causes effort angina, followed by unstable angina, followed by a heart attack. (See Figure 5.) Unfortunately, much of the time this does not happen. Atherosclerosis does not behave the same in each patient. It doesn't grow at the same rate in every person, and it does not cause the same type of blockage in every person.

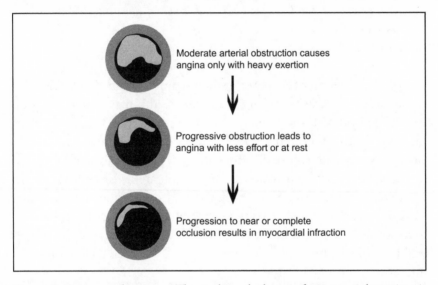

Moderate arterial obstruction causes angina only with heavy exertion

Progressive obstruction leads to angina with less effort or at rest

Progression to near or complete occlusion results in myocardial infraction

Figure 5: Coronary obstruction. The traditional theory of coronary obstruction in atherosclerosis, now known to be wrong in most cases of acute blockage of the arteries. Slow progression of plaque to complete obstruction is much less common than rupture of a small plaque with formation of a blood clot as a cause of heart attack.

Challenges to the Traditional View

I fainted during a tennis match, and was taken to the hospital. They wheeled me in to get an angiogram and wheeled me back out because I needed triple bypass surgery.
Donald D.

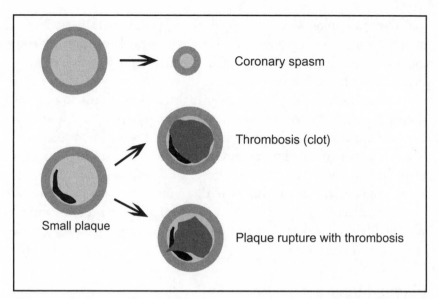

Figure 6: Alternative explanations for acute complete obstruction of coronary arteries. Pure spasm of an artery is rare, and most heart attacks are now known to be caused by blood clots triggered by the rupture of incompletely obstructive plaques.

> *I had some discomfort and muscle weakness on the day before New Year's Eve, 1996. The blood tests came back suggesting that I'd had a heart attack. That night I had dinner with some friends who knew a heart surgeon. I called him, explained the blood test results and he said, "Get over here." They sent an ambulance to pick me up the next morning and did an angioplasty as soon as I arrived. It was during that procedure that they found an additional blockage in a different artery that was much more severe. It was sort of a double wake-up call.*
> *Demetre S.*

There are a number of observations that challenge the traditional view. First, not every person experiences angina in the same way—or at all. In some patients effort angina remains stable and never progresses to unstable angina. Some patients never experience effort angina, and progress straight to unstable angina with no warnings. Some patients suffer a myocardial infarction as the first indication of coronary artery disease. It is well recognized that heart attacks can occur in people who have just had a complete check-up and were told that everything seemed normal. Some people have heart attacks even though a recent exercise test was entirely normal. For these patients, the myocardial infarction itself is often the first—and sometimes fatal—expression of heart disease.

How is this possible? The answer is that a slowly growing occlusion that eventually totally obstructs a coronary artery isn't the only cause of myocardial infarction, and it is not the major reason why heart attacks occur. While narrowing of the coronary arteries puts your circulatory system at risk, the critical link between coronary artery disease and heart attacks is that atherosclerotic plaques that only partially block the artery can undergo abrupt and catastrophic structural changes that lead to complete occlusion (closing) of the artery. (See Figure 6.)

Plaque Rupture

Plaque formations do not always remain stable over time. Some deposits contain more fatty cells and these fatty plaques are prone to rupture, particularly in the presence of high blood pressure. When a plaque deposit ruptures, the cap of the deposit is torn off and debris is released into the blood stream. When this happens, the blood's defense system can mistake this rupture for an internal injury. If so, it will create one or more blood clots to help seal the rupture.

A blood clot is a normal response to injury in the body, including in the blood vessels themselves. It is part of the body's defense against the many injuries that people sustain over the course of their lives. Unfortunately, this proactive system of defense can have unintended consequences. If a blood clot forms in a coronary artery already partially blocked by atherosclerosis, that clot can cut off blood flow to part of the heart muscle.

Coronary Spasm

Another, but far less common, cause of sudden obstruction of the coronary arteries is spasm of a coronary artery. A coronary spasm is the abrupt contraction of one small part of an artery. A spasm may occur in any artery, rarely even in a completely normal artery, but is more likely to occur in an artery that already is partially blocked by arterial plaque. This plaque alters the smooth muscle cells inside the artery wall, making them more apt to contract suddenly with very little stimulus. This can lead to complete obstruction of the artery even in when there is not much underlying plaque. Fortunately, spasm of a coronary artery is extremely rare in people who do not already experience symptoms of severe coronary artery disease. It is characterized by symptoms of reversible angina that do not seem to be related in any way to effort or emotional stress.

What Happens During a Heart Attack?

Every heart attack, referred to medically as a myocardial infarction (MI), differs in terms of what triggers it, how long it lasts, and the damage it leaves behind. In some cases, an MI can be so mild that it causes no symptoms and can only be detected by an ECG or by blood tests that check for the chemical indicators of a heart attack. These are called silent heart attacks. They can be particularly danger-ous because they damage your heart without giving you a warning that something is wrong. Often, they are precursors to larger, more damaging heart attacks.

Here is the sequence of events that occurs in the body during most heart attacks.

You feel pain. Most heart attacks do cause some pain; many cause extreme pain, along with sweating, anxiety, and confusion. The pain may not be the classic squeezing or pressure in the central part of the chest. It can appear in the neck or back, along one arm, or in the elbows. It can even be in the teeth or jaw. Every patient is different and blockages in different arteries may cause varying symptoms. When angina or a heart attack occurs, shortness of breath may be even more prominent than pain.

Your body prepares for trauma. The pain and anxiety of a heart attack activates the body's sympathetic nervous system, the part of the body that controls automatic responses to stimuli. The sympathetic nervous system, also called the "fight-or-flight" response, activates chemicals including adrenaline that prepare the body for confrontation or trauma. Unfortunately, one of the first things the sympathetic nervous system does during an acute heart attack is to make the heart pump harder and faster. This extra activity means that the heart will need even more oxygen, even though one or more of the coronary arteries may be completely blocked. As a result, the cells in the heart will be under further stress as the demand for oxygen continues to increase.

Your blood pressure goes up. The sympathetic nervous system also constricts the major arteries in order to move blood out of less critical areas, such as the bowels, and into more critical areas, such as the muscles and brain. This tends to raise the blood pressure, which can make the plaque in the coronary arteries susceptible to more ruptures. The sympathetic nervous system also activates the blood's clotting system of in preparation for a possible physical injury. All of these factors together can cause multiple plaque ruptures and blockages to occur hours after the original heart attack has begun.

A struggling, weakened heart may not be able to pump blood adequately to key organs, including the kidneys. In response, the kidneys will secrete renin, which will set off a cascade of chemicals to further constrict arteries and retain fluids in a major effort to preserve blood volume and prevent circulatory shock. This sudden, high blood pressure can set off another round of plaque ruptures and blood clots.

In this way a myocardial infarction is an event that continues to evolve. It can have powerful ongoing negative effects on your health long after the event first begins. The medical care you get needs to rapidly address all of these issues. In this context, it is clear why in addition to oxygen and pain relief, immediate treatment to limit the clotting response of the body and to block the activation of the sympathetic nervous system is a cornerstone of treatment of acute heart attacks.

Further treatment is designed to either dissolve the clot chemically, or to remove it and reduce the obstruction via angioplasty and stenting. The sooner the obstructing coronary artery blockage is relieved, the better it is for the heart.

The Importance of Early Medical Attention

A myocardial infarction does not kill all of the cells in the heart. There are several major coronary arteries that supply blood to different sections of the heart, and they can branch off several times into smaller vessels, called collateral arterioles, that can sometimes feed other areas of the heart. An arterial occlusion affects only the heart muscle cells on the far side of the blockage. (See Figure 7.)

During a heart attack, this area may resemble a target. The cells in the center will die first, while the cells around this area may merely become stunned by severe metabolic injury that limits the ability of the cells to contract but does not cause them to die. This inability to contract may persist for some time, even if blood flow to the damaged area is improved. This limited functional recovery of heart muscle cells can happen after frequent and prolonged periods of angina even if you don't have a heart attack. In these cases, the heart muscle cells are actually called "stunned," and when dysfunction is extremely prolonged but ultimately reversible in these cells, they are said to have been "hibernating."

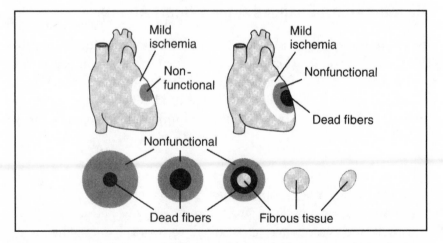

Figure 7: Small and large areas of coronary ischemia, with dead heart muscle cells due to myocardial infarction in the center of the large area that will remain nonfunctional and develop into a scar (fibrous tissue).

That's why getting to the hospital quickly is so crucial. Doctors can take immediate steps to prevent further blood clots, decrease your heart rate and blood pressure to reduce the excess demand of the heart for oxygen, and ideally remove a blockage to restore some blood flow. The faster this happens, the more likely those dormant cells around the infarction are to recover and resume functioning again. This will limit the total amount of damage done to the heart muscle in the course of the heart attack.

Another important reason for getting early medical attention during a heart attack is that the most harmful heart rhythm disturbances generally occur early in the course of muscle damage. The most serious of these irregularities, ventricular fibrillation, is responsible for most of the early death that occurs with heart attacks. Some patients will survive a heart attack but be left with a risk of developing potentially dangerous arrhythmias in the future, even after the initial symptoms are gone and the cell damage has healed. This is more common in people who suffer larger areas of heart tissue damage. Identifying individuals at risk for dangerous arrhythmias is an important aspect of long-term care. If you've had a heart attack you should discuss this issue with your doctor.

How the Heart Changes After a Heart Attack

Scar tissue appears. A severe heart attack can damage a significant number of heart muscle cells. During the healing process, those damaged cells are gradually replaced with scar tissue, which doesn't contract to pump blood. These dead cells may permanently interfere with the ventricle's ability to pump adequate amounts of blood.

The heart muscle thickens. The tissue surrounding the scarred area will be under additional burden to make up for the lost pumping power. Heart muscle is, after all, muscle tissue, and it does what muscle tissue does when it is asked to work harder. That is, it becomes thicker and stronger. This process is called hypertrophy. If the infarcted (damaged) area is small enough, this thicker, stronger tissue around it can fully compensate for the damage.

Classifications of Heart Failure

NY Heart Association's functional classifications of heart failure:

Class I. Patients usually have no symptoms, and no limitations in functional activity.

Class II. Many patients experience mild symptoms that limit strenuous activity.

Class III. At this point patients are noticing marked symptoms that prevent many ordinary activities.

Class IV. Symptoms are noticeable even at rest and are so severe that they are nearly debilitating.

The ventricle dilates. If the infarcted area is too large, the ventricle may be unable to pump out enough blood to feed the body's organs and tissues. As a result, the muscle tissue is likely to stretch and dilate under the pressure of the blood entering the ventricle. This condition sets the stage for heart failure.

What Is Heart Failure?

Heart failure is a progressive condition in which the heart can no longer pump adequate amounts of blood. One way that doctors measure the pumping power of the ventricle is in terms of the percent of the total blood in the chamber that is expelled with each contraction. This is known as the ejection fraction. A normal ventricle pumps out 50 percent to 70 percent of its blood with every contraction. When the ejection fraction is reduced to less than 40 percent, some symptoms of heart failure may occur, but symptoms are more common when the ejection fraction falls below 30 percent.

The heart generally adapts to a reduction of ejection fraction by becoming larger. Having more total blood in the chamber allows a larger volume of blood to be ejected with each weaker contraction. This adaptation can be remarkably effective for a time. Some individuals' hearts can function with remarkably low ejection fractions, perhaps as low as 10 percent, given enough time to enlarge and adapt to progressive damage. But at some point in the course of heart failure, the reduced ability to pump blood will cause blood to pool in the lungs and extremities and lead to swelling of the legs or generalized bloating in the body, along with fatigue and shortness of breath.

When this occurs, the kidneys may respond by hanging on to sodium and fluids, causing further bloating and weight gain. This is the basic protective response of the kidneys whenever their blood flow is interrupted, even though in this case it tends to make the symptoms of heart failure worse. Although these symptoms can be treated by medication, you should know that heart failure is a chronic, progressive condition that has become a major consequence of various forms of heart disease. It is now one of the most common causes of hospitalization in the world.

How Atherosclerosis Affects Other Organs

I can't walk much. I go about 100 yards and my hip and leg starts to ache and when I stop the pain stops. They are 90 percent sure that I have claudication in my leg and that goes along with the atherosclerosis. I don't know what they're going to do about that.
Lou S.

Arteries bring oxygen-rich blood to every major organ in your body, not just the heart. As the atherosclerotic plaque builds in other major arteries, your other organs may also be starved for blood, causing further complications.

The brain. Blockages in the carotid or vertebral arteries result in a reduced blood flow to the brain. When you suffer a temporary lack of oxygen (ischemia) to the brain, it is called a transient ischemic attack (TIA). If this lack of oxygen becomes critical, you may suffer a stroke in which some of the brain cells die. In this context, a TIA is similar to angina, while a stroke is similar to a myocardial infarction.

The kidneys. When the renal arteries, which feed your kidneys, become partially blocked, the kidneys respond by raising your blood pressure and blood volume. The kidneys do this by releasing several

Effects of Atherosclerosis on Target Organs		
	Reversible ischemia	**Irreversible iscemia**
Heart	Angina	Myocardial infarction
Brain	Transient ischemic attack (TIA)	Stroke
Limbs	Claudication	Gangrene

Figure 8: Consequences of reversible and irreversible ischemia in the heart and in the brain and the limbs. Reversible ischemia of the heart is angina pectoris, while irreversible ischemia leads to myocardial infarction (a heart attack).

chemicals to constrict arteries throughout the body and by conserving fluid and sodium to increase blood volume. High blood pressure means that your heart has to work harder to pump blood. Over time, this added effort can stress the heart enough to contribute to heart failure. Further, the kidneys themselves can begin to fail when blood flow becomes limited by atherosclerosis in the renal arteries.

The legs. The muscles and tissues of your legs also receive blood through arteries. Atherosclerosis in these arteries can result in pain known as claudication. Similar to angina, claudication occurs primarily during exercise, when the muscles need extra oxygen that the arteries cannot supply.

Some people experience claudication as muscle weakness or cramping, or as a sensation of cold or numbness in the arms and legs. Over time, the pain may become more constant. People who have diabetes are at much greater risk of developing claudication. If you have claudication, your atherosclerosis has become quite advanced, and as a result you are at much higher risk for suffering a heart attack or stroke. If claudication progresses to the point where the blood flow is cut off long enough, the tissue on the other side of the blockage will die—just as heart tissue dies in a heart attack. This tissue can become infected and, untreated, lead to gangrene in that part of the body.

Some Questions to Ask

Now that you have reviewed the way your heart works, how arterial plaque grows and how it sets the stage for coronary events, you will be able to ask more specific questions of your doctor about the nature of your blockages and what has been done or might be done about them. You can also talk to your doctor about the amount of heart muscle damage you may have suffered, and what long-term issues you may face as your disease progresses. Some specific questions you might ask, are:

* *Do I have significant blockages in my coronary arteries, and if so, in which ones?*

* *Do these blockages affect my left, or front, ventricle, the main pumping chamber of the heart?*

* *Will I need angioplasty or stenting for these blockages in the future?*

* *Did I sustain heart muscle damage during my heart attack? If so, how does this affect my recovery?*

* *Am I at high risk for developing heart failure? If so, what symptoms should I be aware of? What medications and interventions might delay or prevent this outcome?*

Chapter 5

◆ ❖ ◆ ◆ ❖ ◆ ◆ ◆ ❖ ◆ ◆ ❖ ◆ ◆ ◆ ❖ ◆ ◆

Taking the Risk
Factors to Heart
A Summary of the Major
Risk Factors for Heart Disease

Most people are pretty familiar with the accepted major risk factors for heart disease. They have been presented in a great number of ways. Your primary care physician may have talked to you about your risk factors and how to modify them, or you may have read about the factors that can affect your likelihood of developing heart disease.

Now that you have experienced heart problems, you can no longer afford to ignore these risks. So, here they are again, the factors that most influence the course of your heart disease. Although the first two can't be changed, the rest can be modified with lifestyle changes and medications—often with great results.

The fear we have now is for our sons. They refuse to believe that at their young age they can be affected by heart disease. But I know they can be affected. Lou's dad had a heart attack at 52, and Lou had his first at 46. They should be taking steps now to avoid all that we've been through. Denise S.

What Is a Risk Factor?

The first landmark study of the possible causes of heart disease began in 1948, in Framingham, Massachusetts. Researchers decided to conduct a long-term study to try to uncover the connection between heart disease and factors such as lifestyle and heredity. To do this, they randomly selected a group of 5,200 residents of Framingham. The researchers took initial medical histories for these subjects, and then examined them every other year for the rest of their lives.

More than 55 years later the study continues with many of the children and grandchildren of the original participants now enrolled. As such it is one of the most extensive, multi-generational studies of health in medical history. Researchers have published more than 1,000 studies using data from the Framingham Heart Study, as it is known, and it has helped illuminate many of the causes of heart disease.

One of the many contributions the Framingham researchers have made is to the understanding of risk factors. In fact, they were the ones who coined this term to describe characteristics that contribute to cardiovascular disease.

The Risk Factors

The number of risk factors that researchers have identified has grown over the decades, and it continues to change as more research is being done. New risk factors are emerging and will be subject to more research until they can be established. In the meantime, the commonly-accepted list of major risk factors for heart disease now includes:

* *Heredity*
* *Age and sex*
* *Smoking*
* *High cholesterol*
* *Blood sugar*
* *High blood pressure*
* *Sedentary lifestyle*
* *Stress*

Heredity

If your mother or father has heart disease, or if several of your blood relatives have heart disease, then you are at higher risk for developing the condition, even if you feel perfectly healthy. If you have heart disease, then your children are at higher risk, as well.

Age and Sex

The risk of suffering a heart attack increases with age. For men, the risk begins to increase after age 45. For women, risk increases sharply after menopause. Statistically, more men suffer from heart disease than women, but it is a leading cause of death for both genders.

Smoking

This was one of the first links made between lifestyle and disease. Smokers are far more likely to die of heart disease than nonsmokers. Heavy smokers are three to five times as likely to suffer a heart attack as nonsmokers.

Most people know that smoking isn't good for them. Thanks to aggressive public education campaigns the prevalence of smoking among adults in this country has dropped to less than 25 percent since 1965, when approximately 42 percent of adults smoked. This is good news because doctors know that people who smoke are, on average, about 10 years younger than nonsmokers when they have their first heart attack. Smokers also tend to have fewer other risk factors for heart disease when they show up in the emergency room.

What the Research Shows

Researchers discovered the powerful effects of smoking when they followed a group of 2,600 people after their first heart attack. Those who continued to smoke were 50 percent more likely to suffer another heart attack than nonsmokers. Those who quit smoking and stuck with it for three years were no more likely to suffer another event than people who had never smoked.

In addition, your first heart attack is more likely to be fatal if you smoke. This increased risk of immediate death disappears within days of stopping smoking. This in itself should be an incentive to quit. Unfortunately, many people don't quit, even after their first heart attack—a decision that compounds their health problems.

Cholesterol

At first, researchers noticed a correlation between high total cholesterol and coronary mortality. Now, they understand that the relationship is more complex because there are different types of cholesterol. A high level of LDL particles or "bad" cholesterol encourages the progression of heart disease; HDL or "good" cholesterol has a protective effect, so a low level of this substance increases risk.

Reducing cholesterol, and specifically reducing LDL cholesterol, has profoundly beneficial effects on your likelihood of suffering a heart attack or stroke. In recent decades, researchers have discovered that cholesterol is a primary cause of the development of arterial plaque, and that the more arterial plaque you have, the more likely you are to suffer from a potentially heart attack or stroke.

What the Research Shows

In the Multiple Risk Factor Intervention Trial, researchers measured the cholesterol levels of 356,222 men who had no previous history of heart disease. After six years of follow-up, researchers discovered that in each age group, higher total cholesterol correlated directly with coronary death. The risk increased at a level above 200 mg/dl of cholesterol. In fact, those men with a total cholesterol count that was at or near 244 mg/dl were more than twice as likely to die of heart disease in the six-year follow-up than those with a total cholesterol level below 182 mg/dl. Men with cholesterol levels above 245 mg/dl were nearly 3.5 times more likely to die than those with low cholesterol. Once you have heart disease, lowering your cholesterol becomes even more important.

Choose Your Poison

Look at the nutritional content of any fast food menu item and you would be tempted to think that the four major food groups are calories, fat, cholesterol, and sodium. Here are some examples from a typical fast food menu.

Breakfast sandwich: 480 calories; 30 grams fat; 245 milligrams cholesterol; 1300 milligrams sodium.

Hamburger: 450 to 550 calories; 20 to 35 grams fat; 75 to 85 milligrams cholesterol; 780 milligrams sodium.

French fries: 320 calories; 3 grams fat; 210 milligrams cholesterol; 40 milligrams sodium.

The best way to eliminate the risk that high cholesterol poses is to reduce the cholesterol circulating in your blood. The first step is to change your diet. If that doesn't work, you may also have to take cholesterol-lowering medication.

However, making the type of lifestyle changes necessary to accomplish this is difficult to do. A number of years ago, it was estimated that 80 percent of Americans live within three miles of the leading fast food chain. Many, if not most, busy people rely on fast food or takeout food several times a week as an alternative to grocery shopping and cooking at home. One look at the fat and cholesterol content of fast food restaurant fare will tell you why high cholesterol is such a problem for so many adults. In recent years, fast food chains have made more of an effort to offer heart healthy choices, but you benefit from these efforts only if choose the healthier options.

Blood Sugar

Researchers are beginning to recognize that glucose is a cardiovascular risk factor similar to blood pressure and cholesterol. This means that higher levels confer higher risk. Sugar, or glucose, is meant to circulate only briefly in the blood stream, until insulin can convert it into a fuel that cells can store and use later. If it circulates for too long it has a number of destructive effects on the body. First, it damages blood vessels of every size. This is particularly dangerous in the delicate vascular beds of the retina and the kidneys, but it is equally destructive to larger arteries and arterioles, where along with high levels of insulin it encourages the oxidation of LDL particles and the accumulation of arterial plaque.

Patients who have diabetes and heart disease need to be extra vigilant about controlling their fasting glucose levels in order to reduce their chances of suffering a heart attack or stroke. If you have type 1 diabetes, this means careful monitoring of your insulin dosage to optimize glucose control. If you have type 2 diabetes, this means strictly controlling your diet, making sure you get exercise, and perhaps taking oral anti-diabetic agents to further increase your body's sensitivity to insulin. In both cases, the goal is to bring fasting glucose level to near-normal values. Overall control of sugar metabolism is also estimated by testing for glycosylated hemoglobin (HbA1C) levels. This measurement reflects the average sugar level of the blood over a longer period of time. Healthy HbA1C levels should be below 6.5 percent.

Sedentary Lifestyle

Exercise helps protect your cardiovascular system from disease. It improves circulation, and boosts the blood's oxygen content. It encourages the body to produce chemicals that dilate arteries, and it burns the sugar and fat that might otherwise circulate long enough to become arterial plaque.

Studies show that although the risk of mortality is very high among absolute couch potatoes, this risk drops sharply with just a slight increase in exercise. Even if you have never exercised before, you can dramatically improve your level of fitness with only modest effort. In fact, exercise capacity tends to show the most improvement among people who have no experience with exercise. This applies equally to people in nearly every age group.

What the Research Shows

In 1984 a group of researchers studied 361 patients who had recently suffered heart attacks or had undergone bypass surgery. The patients were grouped according to age and then followed through a 12-week cardiac exercise program. After 12 weeks, researchers found that patients between the ages of 40 and 64 showed an improvement of 48 percent in exercise capacity and a decrease in heart rate and blood pressure of 17 percent. Patients over the age of 65 showed similar results—a 53 percent increase in the amount of exercise they could do and an 18 percent reduction in heart rate and blood pressure.

In the Aerobics Center Longitudinal Study, researchers gave tread-mill exercise tests to 13,334 men and women, and then divided them into five groups according to their fitness levels. Researchers followed these subjects for an average of eight years and found that the least physically fit were almost twice as likely to die as the most physically fit. When researchers considered the causes of death, they found that the individuals with the lowest fitness levels were five times as likely to die of coronary causes as those who were the most physically fit. Physically fit people had fewer cancer deaths, as well.

High Blood Pressure

Doctors once believed that high blood pressure was a natural byproduct of aging. Researchers now know that it is the result of many factors. Some of these factors are genetic and some are caused by diet and stress. At higher levels, blood pressure contributes to heart disease by damaging arteries and encouraging strokes and blood clots. It is increasingly recognized that (like cholesterol) the lower the blood pressure level, the less the risk.

Many large studies have shown that high blood pressure is more associated with risk of stroke than risk of heart attack. However, in people with coronary disease untreated hypertension causes

---

What the Research Shows

To determine the effect of high blood pressure on risk of coronary artery disease, researchers pooled the results of nine earlier studies on elevated diastolic blood pressure. The studies included information on 420,000 subjects who were followed for 10 years. Researchers found that the people who had the highest level of diastolic blood pressure (105 mm Hg) were 10 to 12 times more likely to suffer a stroke as those with the lowest level (76 mm Hg). Patients at that highest level were also five to six times more likely to develop heart disease than those at the lowest level. Further, they found that the incidence of heart disease and stroke increased steadily as diastolic blood pressures increased. In other words, every 7.5 mm Hg increase in diastolic blood pressure represented a 46 percent increase in the risk of stroke and a 29 percent increase in the risk of heart disease.

---

atherosclerosis to build in all of the arteries of the body, including those in the heart.

More recent studies have now shown similar increments in risk of stroke and heart disease with elevations of systolic pressure and pulse pressure, particularly in the elderly. The Joint National Committee on Prevention, Detection, Evaluation, and Treatment of High Blood Pressure recently reported that systolic blood pressure over 140 mm Hg is a more potent risk factor than diastolic pressure. The risk of future cardiovascular disease just about doubles for every 20 mm rise in systolic blood pressure over 115 mm Hg, so (just as with cholesterol levels) lower is better.

Stress

In addition to studying risk factors that contribute to the ongoing development of heart disease, researchers have also looked at things that can bring on a sudden cardiac event. One of the most profound discoveries in this area is that episodes of extreme anger and stress can trigger heart attacks.

What the Research Shows

Researchers have paid particular attention to people who experience frequent episodes of rage. One group of researchers interviewed 1305 men with an average age of 61 who had no symptoms of coronary heart disease. These men completed a questionnaire to determine how well or poorly an individual can control his or her anger, called the Minnesota Multiphasic Personality Inventory (MMPI-2). Over seven years of follow-up, researchers discovered that men who reported the highest propensity for anger were more than three times as likely to be diagnosed with heart disease or to suffer a heart attack than those with the lowest tendency toward anger. In addition, men whose inclination to get angry fell in the middle of the range were still twice as likely to develop heart disease or a heart attack as those at the low end of the scale.

In a similar study, researchers interviewed 1,623 men and women a few days after their heart attack. The patients answered two questionnaires to determine how frequently they experience episodes of anger and how many triggering factors they experienced in the days before their heart attacks. Researchers found that patients were more than twice as likely to suffer a heart attack within two hours of having an outburst of anger. Researchers further inquired about the regular use of low-dose aspirin and found that those who took aspirin regularly had a much lower risk of suffering a heart attack after an episode of anger. By contrast, those who did not take aspirin every day were almost three times as likely to suffer a heart attack after being angry.

For decades, doctors have been telling heart patients to take it easy, and to try to avoid situations that might be particularly upsetting. In the past two decades, researchers have isolated a real link between triggers such as physical exertion, sexual activity, anger, and stress, and the onset of angina and heart attacks. In 1991, researchers interviewed heart attack survivors and found that a heart attack is more than twice as likely to occur within three hours of waking up in the morning. That is a time of day when your heart rate and blood pressure naturally accelerate, and even that small change can set the stage for a coronary event. For people with heart disease, daily stressful activities such as driving in heavy traffic, arguing with co workers or spouses, or dealing with the pressure of a deadline can also serve as triggers for heart attacks and strokes.

How do stress and anger put you in so much danger? Tension and anger rapidly increase your heart rate and blood pressure. An increase in heart rate can increase the heart's need for oxygen, while an increase in arterial resistance—or blood pressure—can reduce the available supply of blood to the heart and major organs. In the presence of atherosclerosis, which narrows arteries and partially blocks blood flow, this increased need for oxygen and concurrent decrease in its supply can cause the cells in your heart to suffer a critical lack of oxygen. If the lack of oxygen is severe enough, an episode of angina or a heart attack may follow. If this high blood pressure also injures an artery or ruptures an accumulation of unstable plaque, it can also trigger blood clots, leading to a heart attack.

In light of this information, your doctor may advise you to relax and lighten up—and to take a low dose of aspirin or some other antiplatelet medication every day. Changing your outlook won't necessarily be easy. Some people are as addicted to anger and stress as others are to cigarettes or junk food. Learning to let go of anger and stress are difficult ongoing challenges, but for people with heart disease, they yield significant benefits.

Your Prevention Goals

In the next several years, your goal has to be to reduce or eliminate as many risk factors as you can. Reducing your risk factors is the key to improving your survival and preserving your quality of life. You may even be able to reverse your heart disease if you work diligently to modify your risk factors.

Important research will be published in the next several years that explores emerging risk factors such as lipoprotein (a) (called "lipoprotein little a"), C-reactive protein, and homocysteine.

Cumulative Risk Reduction

Your total risk for having another heart attack is the product of separate risk factors. Risk and risk reduction are cumulative, meaning that the more risk factors you have, the more likely you are to suffer a heart attack. Conversely, the more steps you take to reduce your risk, the less likely you will be to have a heart attack. Consider a hypothetical situation in which each risk factor actually doubles the likelihood of a coronary event. In this setting, reducing just some of your risk factors can substantially reduce your total heart disease risk, even if other factors do not change.

Number of doubling risk factors:	1	2	3	4	5	6
Cumulative relative risk:	2x	4x	8x	16x	32x	64x

Elimination of one risk factor can reduce your total cardiac risk by 50 percent. Elimination of two factors can reduce your risk by 75 percent.

Emerging Risk Factors

Two new substances, C-reactive protein and homocystein, are currently being studied to determine if they have any value in predicting coronary risk.

C-reactive protein (CRP). This is a chemical produced by the liver when you have an infection or chronic inflammation. Biological researchers have known about this substance for many years, but they are now studying its possible link with heart disease. Doctors now know that people with heart disease often have an elevated level of CRP in their blood. In fact, having a high level of CRP in your blood means that you are at increased risk of suffering a coronary event. The question is whether atherosclerosis is the cause

Hormone Replacement Therapy

It has been recognized for years that atherosclerotic disease in women tends to occur at a later age than it does in men. Because arterial disease, including coronary artery disease, seems to accelerate in women after menopause, it was long suspected that younger women were protected from atherosclerosis by estrogen and progesterone, the female hormones. Several decades ago, some doctors gave estrogen to men after a cardiac event to try to reduce future problems. This experiment didn't work out as anticipated—the men had more, not fewer, cardiac problems while taking estrogen.

But women are different from men, and until quite recently, hormone replacement therapy (HRT) had many theoretically attractive potential benefits for postmenopausal women. In addition to protecting the heart from infarction and the brain from strokes after menopause, HRT should retard the development of osteoporosis. By strengthening bones, HRT should reduce the serious problem of hip fracture in older women. Unfortunately, the promise of improved vascular health with HRT has not been supported by recent large scale controlled studies. In the Heart and Estrogen/progesterone Replacement Study (HERS), combined estrogen and progesterone therapy in postmenopausal women was not beneficial over placebo after nearly seven years, and it was actually associated with increased heart attacks and blood clots in the veins of the legs and in the lungs during the first year. Similarly, the Women's Health Initiative (WHI) also found no benefit of combined estrogen/progesterone HRT on survival in women, but rather unexpected increases in rates of heart attack, stroke, blood clots, and breast cancer.

Note that the greatest risk for blood clots with HRT in some of these studies appears to be early, so if you have been on HRT for many years without complications, continuing this therapy may not put you at greater risk. This is something you should discuss with your doctor. Studies on estrogen replacement therapy alone, without additional progesterone, are continuing and you should watch for these results. However, at present, it is the general consensus of the cardiology community that HRT is not effective or safe for the prevention of heart disease.

of an elevated CRP level, or whether that elevated CRP level somehow causes arterial plaque to form. A third possibility is that they are both unrelated consequences of other factors.

At present, there is no reason to request a CRP test from your cardiologist. Currently, doctors aren't even sure that CRP levels can be effectively lowered in people. Even if and when an effective means is developed to lower CRP, there's no guarantee that having a lower level will reduce your risk of heart disease. Future research will surely clarify all of this. In the meantime, your doctor will probably focus on your modifiable risk factors.

Homocysteine. This is an amino acid, a byproduct of the breakdown of another amino acid, called methionine. High levels of homocysteine in the blood have been associated with blood clots and the accelerated accumulation of arterial plaque. These high levels also seem to correlate with high stress and vitamin deficiencies, especially of folic acid (folate) and vitamin B12. These vitamins help break down homocysteine in the blood to make it harmless.

Even if you don't have an actual vitamin deficiency, you can reduce your homocysteine level by taking large doses of folate, along with B6 and B12. It makes sense that the use of these vitamins could reduce cardiac events in people, and many doctors do suggest vitamins to patients with atherosclerosis. However, although it is clear that a high homocysteine level is a risk factor, and that it can be lowered by treatment, no clear studies have shown that lowering it will prevent heart attacks. You may already be taking folate, and since it is potentially helpful, cheap, and without important known side effects, there is no reason not to. Whether you take folate or not, you need to watch for future developments as studies are done to clarify this.

Reversing Your Heart Disease

By modifying as many risk factors as you can, you will drastically reduce your chances of suffering further complications of heart disease. In some cases, people are even able to reverse the progression of heart disease. With exercise, a healthy diet, and in some cases, the right medications, patients can improve blood flow and slow or even reverse the progress of atherosclerosis.

Throughout this book you'll read about a lot of studies in which researchers have found significant decreases in the risk of having a heart attack or stroke in the presence of a medication or lifestyle change. For example, a daily low-dose of aspirin has been shown to reduce risk of a subsequent heart attack by 30 percent. Numerous studies have shown that reducing your cholesterol level by 10 percent can reduce your risk of a subsequent heart attack by 20 percent. You'll read about other studies showing similarly significant changes in risk brought on by exercise and blood pressure control, as well as the use of medications such as beta-blockers and ACE inhibitors.

All of this sounds exciting, and it is. Evaluate all of these statistics and you might be tempted to believe it would be impossible for you to have a heart attack or stroke or need a revascularization procedure if you just make the right choices. Of course, that's not true. The numbers cited in the studies refer to population statistics. A 30 percent reduction in relative risk means that in any study, of the 100 people who would have been expected to suffer a heart attack, 30 did not. The other 70 took the pill or modified the risk factor and had a heart attack anyway. Individual consequences are actually all or none, but you do want the odds on your side.

Your individual risk is yours alone and it depends in part on many factors that you can't change, such as your heredity and your age, as well as risk factors that are still unknown or can't yet be modified. Reducing your risk by 80 percent means that you still have a 20 percent risk of having a heart attack, not that you're only likely to get 20 percent of a heart attack. Still, an 80 percent reduction in risk is highly significant; it can result in a striking improvement in your overall health and in the quality of your life.

Ultimately, one of the greatest achievements in the field of coronary care over the past 40 years has been the identification of risk factors and the development of methods for modifying them. Not only do cardiologists and surgeons have many more tools and techniques at hand to help patients in acute distress, but doctors can also teach patients specific ways to change the trajectory of their disease. The more you know about heart disease and the interventions available to you, the more likely you are to take an active role in managing your own recovery.

Some Questions to Ask

Before you read further about the causes of heart disease and the interventions designed to protect you against further complications, you may want to stop and consider what your own risk factors are. Some of these risk factors, such as age, gender, and heredity, can't be changed. Most others can be changed in order to improve your health and slow the progression of your disease. Gathering information about your risk factors is an important step in taking charge of your health. Some questions you may want to consider are:

* *Am I a smoker? If so, am I ready to quit?*

* *What is my cholesterol level and what can I do to reduce it?*

* *Do I exercise? How can I add exercise to my daily routine?*

* *How much of a role does stress play in my life and how can I reduce that stress?*

* *What are my blood sugar levels? If I have diabetes, am I adequately controlling my blood sugar?*

* *What is my blood pressure? Is it too high and if so, what can I do to lower it?*

* *Am I taking hormone replacement therapy and if so, is it appropriate?*

* *Do I take a multi-vitamin rich in folic acid?*

◆ ◆ ❖ ◆ ◆ ❖ ◆ ◆ ❖ ◆ ◆ ❖ ◆ ◆ ❖ ◆ ◆ ❖ ◆ ◆ ❖ ◆ ◆ ❖

The next few chapters describe certain drugs whose value has been proven to improve survival in multiple large-scale studies. Does this mean you should be taking all of these drugs?

Maybe, but every patient is different. A patient who has had an angioplasty and stent for angina, who has no evidence of further coronary blockages, is different from a patient with a heart attack who has stable angina after the event. A patient with normal pumping power of the heart is different from a patient with a weak heart. Some of these recommendations are especially effective for people who have had heart attacks, while others are more helpful for people with angina. Others were developed for people who don't yet have heart disease. As a result, each of the interventions you will read about may not have the same degree of benefit for you.

For some people, particularly those who have survived a heart attack, certain combinations of drugs work well together to reduce risk. With some exceptions, American Heart Association guidelines recommend for these people the combined use of:

* *anti-platelet drugs (such as aspirin)*
* *beta-blockers*
* *angiotensin blocking drugs*
* *and lipid-lowering agents (drugs to lower cholesterol)*

PART II

◆ ❖ ◆ ◆ ◆ ❖ ◆ ◆ ◆ ❖ ◆ ◆ ◆ ❖ ◆ ◆ ◆ ❖ ◆ ◆ ◆ ❖ ◆ ◆

Commonly Prescribed
Medications for Heart Disease

Some cardiologists extend this principle to other groups of individuals, such as those who have had angioplasty and stenting, while others don't. If you have been completely revascularized by angioplasty or by surgical bypass, and there is no angina, your doctor may not think that all of these medications are necessary. Or your doctor might feel that these drugs can reduce the progression of atherosclerosis, and can therefore be of benefit to you. It's okay to ask pointed questions about why your doctor does or does not think you should take a certain medication.

Studies on new drugs and on combinations of drugs that bear on your personal medical situation will continue to appear in the future. Get your doctor's opinion on what drugs and combinations are right for you. Know your medications, their doses, and their effects. This is where an understanding of the principles underlying drug effects in cardiac patients helps you to work most effectively for your own benefit with your own doctor.

Chapter 6

◆ ◆ ❖ ◆ ◆ ❖ ◆ ◆ ❖ ◆ ◆ ❖ ◆ ◆ ❖ ◆ ◆ ❖ ◆ ◆

Aspirin and Other Anti-Clotting Medications

An Important Step to Prevent a Heart Attack

By far, the most commonly prescribed heart medication is aspirin, the same stuff you probably keep in your medicine cabinet. That's because for most people a low, daily dose of aspirin is a safe and inexpensive way to prevent blood clots that can trigger heart attacks or cause c omplications after angioplasty. Aspirin has several important benefits for people who have heart disease, but it is not for everyone.

Those who can't take aspirin may be able to take other, similar drugs, called antiplatelet medications. Others will be better off taking anticoagulants, which work in a different way to prevent blood clots. People at very high risk of blood clots may wish to take a combination of drugs to reduce their blood's clotting time. Ultimately, for most people with heart disease, eliminating the threat of blood clots is a crucial first step in preventing future heart attacks.

One night I got home from work, cleaned up the house, made dinner, took a shower, poured myself a glass of wine and sat down. Then my throat and ears got sore. I thought, what is this? Then my jaw got in the act. It felt like my teeth were being pulled out. I knew something was wrong, so I took a couple of aspirin. My brother was home, so I asked him to take me to the hospital. I didn't think I was having a heart attack, but I took the aspirin anyway. It turns out I was having a heart attack. Marcy G.

What Does Aspirin Do?

By now, most people know that taking a couple of adult aspirin at the first symptoms of a heart attack can help reduce the seriousness of the heart attack by decreasing the tendency of blood to clot inside arteries. Medical professionals often give aspirin to patients who arrive at the emergency room with symptoms of unstable angina or a myocardial infarction before any other treatment begins.

As well they should.

How is it possible that an ordinary household pain reliever can do all of this? For more than 100 years, aspirin has been sold simply as a pain reliever and anti-inflammatory medication. In the past two decades, however, researchers have discovered that aspirin also acts on the blood in a unique way. It slightly alters the platelets circulating in the blood stream, and by doing so, it prevents them from doing what they do best: promoting the clotting of blood.

Platelets Build Blood Clots

Blood is made up of three major types of cells: red blood cells, which carry oxygen; white blood cells, which fight infection and participate in inflammation; and platelets, which protect the body and the blood vessels themselves against physical injury. Platelets spend most of their time passing innocuously through the body, skimming vessel walls looking for signs of damage. When they pass over a wound—a rupture, tear, or cut in a blood vessel—they stick to the area of injury and release chemicals that reduce local damage and help start the repair process. These chemicals cause the vessel wall to constrict and reduce blood flow to that vessel in order to form a temporary, natural tourniquet while the body addresses the injury further.

They also stimulate more platelets to stick together to form a temporary plug over the injury site. Over time, the plug tightens and seals the wound while the body conducts its repairs.

All of these are steps in the circulatory system's very efficient system for healing itself and for healing the body in response to injury. In a different technological age, when people suffered serious injuries every day, when they used primitive tools to hunt for food, or routinely used hand-to-hand combat to defend themselves, or spent many hours a day carrying out punishing and often dangerous physical labor, the blood's aggressive system of clotting defense against injury was ideal.

These days, people drive everywhere, have sedentary jobs, watch a lot of TV, and eat meals comprised of highly processed, prepackaged foods filled with salt and fat. If you live for several decades in these conditions, the body's system of repairing injuries is quite possibly one of the things that is going to try to kill you. Here's how:

Plaque Triggers Blood Clots

Just as the walls of a blood vessel can tear from an injury, so can the plaque that has built up on arterial walls. In fact, the more advanced the atherosclerosis is, the more likely it is that areas of heavy plaque buildup will become unstable. Some researchers theorize that the growing blockage changes the pattern of blood flow through the vessels in the same way that silt deposits disrupt the flow of water in a fast moving stream. This turbulent blood flow increases the pressure against the artery walls. Eventually, some small spike in blood pressure or in wall stress may cause the plaque to rupture. It could be that quick dash up the stairs to catch a ringing phone, or the frustration of being stuck in traffic. It could be nothing identifiable at all.

When this plaque does rupture, even when the tear is quite small, the blood's defense system treats it as a potentially dangerous injury and begins to create a clot around it. As more and more platelets are attracted to the site of the rupture, the blood clot will continue to grow in size. In some cases, it can ultimately cut off blood flow in the artery.

How Aspirin Works

A couple of decades ago, researchers discovered that aspirin permanently inactivates the enzyme that enables platelets to stick together. This effect on the enzyme lasts for the lifetime of the platelet, meaning that in a quick and generally benign way, aspirin stops blood clots that are promoted by platelets at their source. Aspirin, through other mechanisms, also has some weak effect in reducing the generation of thrombin in the blood, which is another chemical that promotes blood clotting.

When does aspirin do all of this? Almost immediately. Studies have shown that a single adult aspirin (325 mg) can affect the blood platelets and reduce the amount of thrombin in the blood within two hours.

How effective is it in preventing future heart attacks? Very. In one study which looked at the combined results of six trials (6300 patients), daily doses of aspirin less than or equal to 325 mg reduced all-cause mortality by 18 percent. It reduced the number of strokes by 20 percent. Myocardial infarctions were reduced by 30 percent, and other "vascular events" were reduced by 30 percent.

Aspirin also has long-term benefits. Patients who have been prescribed aspirin have significantly higher survival rates 10 years after being discharged from the hospital.

What Is the Correct Dose?

When people take aspirin for a headache, fever, or other body pain, the usual dose is two full size tablets of 325 mg each. However, aspirin has a significant impact on platelets and blood clotting in doses far smaller than a single full-size tablet. A considerable body of research suggests that for many people, aspirin works most effectively in low doses. This is why many doctors use only 81 mg of aspirin daily.

Others believe that platelets in patients with atherosclerosis are more resistant to the effect of aspirin and recommend a full tablet each day. Still other doctors recommend using a 325-mg tablet every other day or three times a week as a compromise between

What the Research Shows

The first study to test aspirin's effectiveness in treating acute heart attacks showed that people given a dosage of aspirin equal to half an adult tablet within 24 hours after symptoms appear, and then every day afterward for five weeks were 23 percent less likely to suffer cardiovascular death, 49 percent less likely to suffer another nonfatal infarction, and 46 percent less likely to suffer a stroke than the control group. These benefits extended equally to women and men. The aspirin was not associated serious side effects involving bleeding, such as hemorrhagic ulcer or stroke.

these regimens. But this routine is harder to keep track of than an every day dose. In any case, higher doses of aspirin than this might produce an adverse balance of effects and at present are not advisable.

What If You Miss a Dose?

One of the problems with other oral anticoagulants has been what doctors call a "rebound effect." These other anticoagulants, sometimes described as "blood thinners," successfully suppress the body's production of thrombin, an enzyme needed to make blood clots. The problem comes when you stop taking an anticoagulant, as you might after surgery or to speed healing from a significant wound or infection. The body begins to work extra hard to make up for all that missing thrombin, which places some patients at a higher short-term risk for developing blood clots.

Aspirin works differently. It affects individual platelets over the course of their entire existence, which is about eight to 12 days. You need to keep taking aspirin because the body is continually replacing those old platelets with new ones. About 10 percent of the blood's platelets are replaced from the bone marrow every day. Halting your aspirin therapy won't make your platelets suddenly more inclined to clot. Rather, the effect of the last dose will gradually diminish as new, unaffected platelets begin to circulate.

Therefore, the effect of missing just a single dose is generally not important, and you can continue with the next regularly scheduled dose without taking a "make-up" pill.

Complications of Aspirin

Despite its many benefits, aspirin also has some risks. The first and most common side effect associated with aspirin is gastrointestinal upset. This symptom may signal a much more serious condition, such as perforation or ulceration of the stomach lining, or internal bleeding. In fact, patients taking as much as 325 mg a day are more than twice as likely to suffer an incident of gastrointestinal tract bleeding.

Most of these incidents are minor. However, large bleeding incidents do occasionally occur from aspirin use, particularly in people who have unsuspected ulcers or a predisposition to developing ulcers. These incidents are much more dangerous because they can abruptly decrease blood volume and cause shock. These serious events are uncommon, and are even less likely to occur when you are taking smaller doses of aspirin.

Unfortunately, while aspirin is preventing blood clots, and therefore lessening your risk of the major kind of stroke, it is also increasing your chances of having another, fortunately less common, kind of stroke: the hemorrhagic stroke. Although the actual rate of hemorrhage associated with low dosages of aspirin is small, the risk is greatest among people who have suffered hemorrhagic stroke in the past or are at high risk of having a burst blood vessel in the brain. People with an aneurysm in an artery in the brain, which is a bulge in the artery that weakens the artery wall and may cause it to burst or bleed, are at increased risk for hemorrhagic stroke. People with these conditions should consult their doctor and weigh the risks of aspirin use against the potential benefits.

Because aspirin successfully interferes with blood clotting, you may need to stop taking it before most major surgical procedures since it will interfere with the body's natural ability to heal. Tell your doctor or dentist that you are taking a daily dose of aspirin well in advance of any surgical procedure or medical test. You may be advised to stop taking aspirin five to 10 days before the procedure.

Who Shouldn't Take Aspirin?

As helpful as it is for prevention of complications of atherosclerosis, for certain people the benefits of aspirin may be outweighed by the risks. For example, your doctor will not prescribe aspirin if you have an aspirin allergy. In other situations, the risk and benefit of aspirin therapy need to be discussed with your doctor, especially if you:

* *Suffer from stomach pains, stomach ulcers, chronic heartburn, or other gastrointestinal disorders that could lead to bleeding.*
* *Have some types of aspirin-sensitive asthma.*
* *Have uncontrolled high blood pressure which could cause a bleeding type of stroke.*
* *Are temporarily at high risk for internal bleeding from a recent injury or operation.*
* *Are unusual in that your platelets are not altered by aspirin.*
* *Suffer from diabetic retinopathy, a serious condition affecting the blood vessels of the eye.*

Drugs That Interfere with Aspirin

Other anti-inflammatory drugs, such as naproxyn or ibuprofen, can partially block the anti-clotting effect of aspirin because they compete for the same receptor site on the platelet. The severity of this interference depends on how often you take these drugs. If you use them every day, you may want to find an alternative anti-inflammatory agent, or if not possible, your doctor may want to discuss your switching to an aspirin alternative.

Aspirin Alternatives

For people who can't tolerate aspirin or who require other methods of platelet inhibition, some alternatives are available.

I take aspirin every day, and I'm on clopidogrel, Normally they try to drop the prescription after 30 to 40 days, but I've had problems with several

stents. The pills are very expensive. That's the one problem. It's getting more expensive all the time.
Jeff G.

Clopidogrel (Trade Name Plavix)

How it works. Platelet stickiness can be stimulated by a number of chemical interactions. For example, platelets also clump together as a reaction to a chemical known as ADP at the site of an injury or perceived injury. While aspirin works by inhibiting an enzyme within the platelet, clopidogrel works by blocking the platelet's ability to respond to ADP. Because these two medications affect platelets differently, clopidogrel and aspirin are sometimes combined for increased anti-platelet effectiveness.

Like aspirin, clopidogrel also works quickly. A 300 mg to 400 mg loading dose of clopidogrel begins reducing blood clotting within two to six hours. After this loading dose, it is effective in smaller doses, such as 75 mg a day. It also seems to be less likely than aspirin to cause gastrointestinal bleeding and upset stomach. Unfortunately, this drug is far more expensive than aspirin, costing in the range of $3 per tablet.

Who should take it? This medication is often prescribed to patients who can't take aspirin, or who have had a heart attack while taking aspirin. It has become increasingly used in addition to aspirin

---

Older Patients

Several recent studies have pointed out that people over the age of 65 are routinely underprescribed a host of heart medications, including aspirin. One possible explanation for this phenomenon is that the older you get, the more likely you are to have had some complication or serious side effect of temporary or chronic aspirin use. However, aspirin is as effective and important in older patients as it is in younger patients with atherosclerotic disease.

A Special Warning

Regular use of the newer, highly effective COX-2 inhibitor class of anti-inflammatory drugs, such as Vioxx (rofecoxib) and Celebrex (celecoxib), should be discussed with your doctor. It turns out that these drugs inhibit a chemical inside the platelet (called cyclo-oxygenase) that helps platelets form blood clots. It also has the theoretical potential to reduce the production of prostacyclin, which helps arteries to dilate. This could be harmful to cardiac patients. So far, the evidence of this effect is not yet definitive, but you will want to follow the evidence about this as additional studies are reported.

---

after coronary angioplasty and stenting, and at present it is used, together with aspirin, in nearly all patients with stents.

Side effects. According to guidelines from the American Heart Association and the American College of Cardiology, clopidogrel is preferable to ticlopidine (brand name Ticlid), another platelet ADP receptor blocker, for patients who are sensitive to aspirin. Ticlopidine has been associated with rare cases of severe loss of multiple blood forming elements. The side effects of clopidogrel can include rash, diarrhea, dyspepsia, excessive bruising, or red spots on the skin. Less common side effects include nosebleeds, or vomiting of dried blood that looks like coffee grounds. Clopidogrel can also be associated with gastrointestinal bleeding and cerebral hemorrhage.

Precautions. Like aspirin, clopidogrel prevents the natural clotting of blood, so it can cause exaggerated bleeding if you have an accident or injury, or if you have surgery or dental work. You should tell any doctor or dentist that you are taking this medication well in advance of any test or medical procedure. If you suffer from excessive bruising or bleeding while on this medication, call your doctor.

Clopidogrel Plus Aspirin

If you have a stent, you will probably be given a prescription for both clopidogrel and aspirin. Because stents are metallic they are especially prone to forming clots, particularly in the first 30 days after they have been implanted. This is because presence of a foreign material disrupts the endothelial cells that line the coronary arteries and may mimic an injury. Over time, the endothelial cells grow over the metallic stent, which reduces the subsequent risk of blood clotting. Patients who receive one of the newer drug-eluting stents may be on clopidogrel for three months or longer, since re-endothelialization may be slower in the presence of these drugs.

Patients who have unstable angina, who have had mild heart attacks, or who have had angioplasty may also be prescribed clopidogrel for long-term use in addition to aspirin. In these high-risk groups, a more aggressive combined antiplatelet therapy can offer an advantage over aspirin alone. As more information becomes available on the efficacy of this combination therapy in different conditions, it may become standard for long-term use. But in every case, anticlotting benefits have to be weighed against the risk of dangerous internal bleeding.

Ticlopidine (Trade Name Ticlid)

Ticlopidine also is a platelet ADP receptor blocker, with effects that are similar to clopidogrel. Because of potentially serious side effects, Ticlopidine is now generally restricted to patients who do not respond to clopidogrel. It was commonly used after stent implantation, also in combination with aspirin. This drug requires two doses a day, and it is far more expensive than aspirin.

Side effects. These can include rash, diarrhea, and occasional cases of serious failure of white and red blood cell production by the body. Less common side effects can include hives or ringing in the ears.

Precautions. Patients taking this drug require periodic monitoring of blood cell levels. You will probably need a blood test every two weeks for the first three months of treatment. If you have any signs of serious bleeding or bruising, if your urine or stools are dark and bloody, if you feel suddenly faint or weak, have a fever or other signs of an infection, you should call your doctor. Patients with stomach ulcers, impaired blood clotting, liver disease, blood disease, or serious kidney disease are generally not prescribed ticiclopidine because of these potential side effects.

Anticoagulants

This type of drug, commonly known as a "blood thinner," also interferes with the body's ability to form blood clots. Anticoagulants prevent the body from generating the enzyme thrombin, which helps solidify the clot by converting fibrinogen to fibrin once the platelets aggregated at the injury site. This type of medication is especially helpful in preventing clots in the veins, as opposed to the arteries, because clots within veins are generally not mediated by platelet aggregation.

Warfarin (Trade Name Coumadin)

How it works. Warfarin is a drug that blocks the formation of multiple blood clotting factors that are made in the liver. Warfarin has been used effectively in patients with heart attacks for several decades. More recently, however, it has taken a back seat to aspirin as the first line of defense against arterial blood clots. It is still used effectively for patients who cannot tolerate aspirin.

Who should take it. Warfarin is the best treatment available when an irregular heart rhythm known as atrial fibrillation is present, which can promote the formation of blood clots in the heart that can break out to cause a stroke or other blockage of an artery. It is also widely used to prevent blood clots in the ventricle of the heart that may occur after large heart attacks.

Despite its clinical value and its essential role in the treatment and prevention of these kinds of blood clots, warfarin does have some problems.

One drawback is that warfarin does cause a higher incidence of bleeding than aspirin does. Its effective dose is very unpredictable and might range from 2 mg or less daily to 15 mg or more daily in different people. The dosage requirement of warfarin can change in response to changes in diet, vitamin intake (particularly vitamin K) and other medications. A small change in warfarin dose can result in an anticoagulation effect that is too low to reduce clotting or, alternatively, that is so great as to promote dangerous bleeding. With appropriate monitoring, warfarin is safe and effective. Accordingly, warfarin treatment requires careful regular monitoring of its effect on the clotting system by periodic blood testing. This is generally done with a blood test called the prothrombin time.

Side effects. As with any anticoagulant, the side effects of warfarin can include unusually heavy bleeding from cuts or injuries, nosebleeds, bleeding gums, unusual bruising, or blood in the urine or stool. It may also cause gastrointestinal upset, nausea, or vomiting. If you have any signs of unusual bleeding or internal bleeding while on this drug, contact your doctor immediately.

Precautions. Warfarin is not a one-size-fits-all medication. Its use must be closely monitored by your doctor. This requires regular blood tests to make sure that you have the right amount in your system, to avoid complications such as internal bleeding. If you have surgery of any kind, you'll have to tell your doctor that you are taking warfarin, as you would with any anticoagulant. Your doctor will usually want you to stop taking it before the surgery.

Dietary precautions. Your diet will affect the amount of warfarin you need. Foods rich in vitamin K, such as green leafy vegetables, cauliflower, dairy products, and liver enhance the body's ability to clot the blood. As such, they can counteract the warfarin in your system. Some dietary supplements also contain vitamin K. If you take a multi-vitamin, a vitamin-enhanced protein shake or breakfast bar, you could be elevating your vitamin K level and therefore interfering with warfarin therapy. This usually is not a problem as long as you are consistent in your diet and use of vitamins.

Many drugs and over-the-counter medications can increase or decrease the effect of warfarin, as well. These potential interactions are very important, and all changes in drug regimen need to be discussed with your doctor when you are taking warfarin.

Warfarin Plus Aspirin

Because warfarin and aspirin have slightly different effects on the blood, and combat the problem of clotting from different aspects of the clotting process, researchers have wondered whether the two drugs could be used together in low doses to prevent the reoccurrence of cardiovascular events.

For many years it was considered too dangerous to combine these medications. More recently, it has been recognized that this can be done when separate indications exist for each drug, such as coronary disease and a blood clot in the lung. Whether combined therapy should be routine for patients with atherosclerotic disease requires further evaluation.

Some Questions to Ask

Most people who have been diagnosed with heart disease will already have been told by their doctors to take a low dose of aspirin every day. In fact, many adults over the age of 60 who have several risk factors for heart disease and who can tolerate aspirin already take it. Still, many other individuals have not been told about aspirin or other antiplatelet medications that may be helpful to them. The next time you see your doctor, you may want to discuss these issues in detail. Some questions you may want to ask are:

* *Am I a good candidate for daily aspirin therapy?*
* *Under what conditions should I stop taking aspirin?*
* *If I'm not a good candidate for aspirin, is there another antiplatelet or anticoagulant medication that I can safely take?*
* *How expensive are these drugs?*
* *If I'm taking warfarin or ticlopidine, how often will I have to have my blood tested for clotting time?*
* *Am I at high risk for blood clotting because of a recent angioplasty or surgery?*
* *If so, what combinations of antiplatelet medications will I take?*
* *How long will I be on these medications?*
* *What side effects or complications should I be aware of?*

Chapter 7

◆ ◆ ❖ ◆ ◆ ❖ ◆ ◆ ❖ ◆ ◆ ❖ ◆ ◆ ❖ ◆ ◆ ◆

The Protective Effects of Beta-Blockers
Reducing the Heart's Workload

Emotional stress and physical exertion have long been known as triggers for heart attacks. Yet, it is nearly impossible to avoid emotional stress while leading a normal life, and avoiding exercise is actually detrimental to people with heart disease. So, if you are at high risk for suffering a heart attack, your doctor may prescribe a medication called a beta-blocker to control your heart rate and help prevent stress or exercise from triggering a heart attack.

In this chapter you'll learn how stress can damage your heart muscle before, during, and after a heart attack. You'll also learn how a beta-blocker works to prevent this damage and how it reduces the workload of the heart and how it can improve the flow of oxygen-rich blood to your heart muscle. You'll read about the different types of beta-blocking drugs and which ones may be most appropriate for you. Finally, you'll learn about the side effects and precautions for beta-blocker therapy.

> *My heart rate is naturally rapid. That's why my doctor put me on a beta-blocker.*
> *Margaret G.*

Reducing the Heart's Workload

In the weeks and months following your surgery or your diagnosis, one of the things your doctor will be most concerned about is your heart rate. A rapid heart rate means that your heart is working harder than it should. In combination with limited blood flow to the heart, this development puts you at risk for angina or myocardial infarction (heart attack). It may also aggravate a potentially fatal arrhythmia, such as ventricular tachycardia or ventricular fibrillation.

The force of each heartbeat is also a factor in the heart's workload. When your heart is pounding, it's working harder than normal. If your arteries are constricted and partially blocked by arterial plaque, your ventricles also have to work harder to push blood into them. When the heart is laboring, it needs more oxygen in the form of blood flow, and when you have heart disease, that extra oxygen just isn't available.

If you were to imagine a drug that could reduce the demand of oxygen by the heart, you would want a drug that would slow the heart rate, decrease the excessive force of contraction of each heartbeat, and reduce the pressure against which the heart must eject blood. That's what beta-blockers do. They have revolutionized the management of heart disease by reducing the immediate negative effects of stress and physical exertion on the heart.

The Fight or Flight Response

You may already know that your heart rate does not remain constant in any 24-hour period. It increases when you are active and decreases when you rest. These changes are controlled by your autonomic nervous system, which regulates your involuntary responses to the world. This system has two components that complement each other. The sympathetic nervous system gets your heart rate moving when you get out of bed each day, when you exercise, and when you feel fear or anger. (See Figure 9.) The parasympathetic system does just the opposite. It prepares you for relaxation and sleep. When your parasympathetic system is in charge, your heart rate slows and your

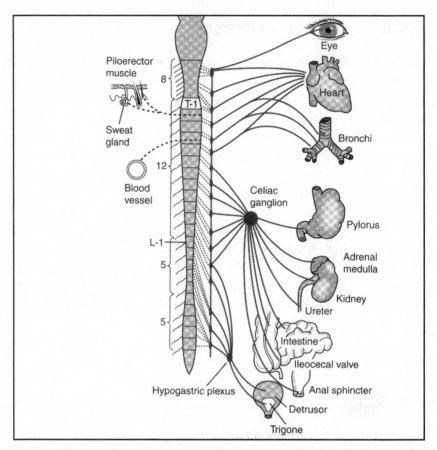

Figure 9: The sympathetic nervous system reaches many organs of the body from branches of the spinal cord, including the heart and the kidneys. Sympathetic stimulation of the body by nerves or by adrenaline released from the adrenal gland readies the body for the "fight or flight" response.

blood pressure goes down as the result of impulses traveling through the parasympathetic nervous system.

Of the two systems, it is the sympathetic nervous system that can cause the most trouble for heart patients. Its primary function is to help your body react to perceived danger. Sometimes called the "fight–or–flight" response, the sympathetic response is activated whenever you feel fear or anger, or during spurts of strenuous exercise. If another car swerves in front of you on your way to work, the sympathetic nervous system instantly prepares you to react by immediately and dramatically modifying most of your body's systems.

The Physical Effects of Stress

The sympathetic response directly stimulates your body's major organs, including the heart, lungs, brain, and liver to mobilize oxygen and energy. Emotional stress and the need for physical action also stimulate these systems by activating chemicals from the adrenal glands, located above the kidneys. These glands secrete a group of chemicals known as catecholamines (adrenaline, also known as epinephrine, is one example) into the blood stream to further prepare the body for stress. Even after the danger has passed, your body needs one to three minutes, and sometimes more, to inactivate these chemicals. Thus, you may have noticed that it takes some time for your heart rate to come down after a real scare or after an episode of anger.

The fight-or-flight response does a number of things to enhance physical performance in times of emergency:

* *It jolts the brain to increase awareness and response time.*
* *It mobilizes glucose and fatty acids in the liver to make more nutrients available to the body.*
* *It encourages the blood to clot in case of injury.*
* *It dilates the bronchiole tubes in the lungs to take in as much oxygen as possible.*

Most important to you, though, is what it does to your circulatory system:

* *It constricts many arteries and capillary beds in an effort to shunt blood to a small number of critical organs and muscles.*
* *It kicks the heart into overdrive.*

These two actions together cause a rapid rise in blood pressure. For example, the sympathetic nervous system can double your heart rate in about ten to fifteen seconds, and double your blood pressure in just as short a time.

These effects take place regardless of the type of stressor involved. The sympathetic nervous system does not really distinguish between a board meeting and a fist fight. It doesn't know the difference between a tense holiday meal and an aerobics class. It simply does everything it can to prepare the body for physical mobility or confrontation whenever it might be called upon.

As a result, in times of emotional or physical stress, the body's circulatory system may be taxed to its limits. Your heart muscle must work harder with less available fuel, while your blood is required to circulate faster and with more force than at any other time. If your circulatory system is already compromised by atherosclerosis, or if your heart muscle has been damaged during a heart attack, this increased demand poses several specific dangers.

A prolonged increase in the heart's workload can cause the starving heart muscle to suffer angina, a myocardial infarction, or even to fibrillate. Over many years, this increased workload can contribute to the development of heart failure.

> *I never believed that stress could ever hurt you physically. But then when we lived in Miami, we had some kittens. It gets so hot sometimes that the kittens crawl up on the tires under your car. One day I was in a hurry and I backed out of the driveway and nearly rolled over one of the kittens. Right after I realized what I had done, I had angina so bad that I was on my knees.*
> *Lou S.*

Sources of Stress

It is no coincidence that so many people suffer heart attacks within the first three hours after awakening. This is when the sympathetic system is most activated. Among people who are employed, there is a somewhat higher risk of suffering a heart attack on a Monday morning. (This cannot be avoided by not working on Mondays or in the mornings—it applies to whenever you return to work after your time off.)

For most heart patients, and in fact most people, acute stress in modern life is only rarely caused by physical confrontation or even by physical exertion. It is caused by perceived danger, emotional fears, and verbal confrontation in both the work and home environments. Many people live in a state of chronic emotional stress and some say they like it that way.

One executive being wheeled into the coronary care unit with a heart attack answered a routine medical question about gastrointestinal symptoms by stating: "I don't get ulcers; I give them." To him, that statement was a measure of his success. He didn't yet understand that chronic activation of the sympathetic nervous system is a primary pathway for heart disease. He didn't know that episodes of anger and hostility are triggers for heart attacks and strokes. Of course these aren't the only triggers. There are many other emotional and physical conditions that predispose patients to an elevated heart rate (see "Factors Contributing to Chronic Sympathetic Activation").

Negative Effects of Stress

An overactive sympathetic nervous system, which is often marked by a resting heart rate at or above 90 beats per minute, has several negative effects on your circulatory system.

The accelerated development of atherosclerosis. When your heart rate and blood pressure rise together, your blood is forced to move faster through your arteries. Over time, the pressure can damage the endothelial cells lining your blood vessels. This occurrence sets off a cascade of reactions that causes the build-up of atherosclerotic plaque.

Coronary spasm. This is a situation in which a portion of an artery abruptly contracts, reducing or shutting off its blood flow. Coronary spasm rarely occurs in completely healthy arteries. Rather, it usually occurs in arteries already partially blocked by atherosclerosis. Spasm of a coronary artery doesn't usually last long enough to cause a heart attack, but it can result in a lengthy episode of unstable angina, which is generally not related to exercise or to emotional stress. Of course, if spasm occurs in an artery severely blocked by arterial plaque or if it occurs along with a blood clot, then it can cut off the blood flow and can cause a heart attack.

Spasm in a coronary artery can be triggered by any number of things, including changes in nervous system activity, elevated blood

---

Factors Contributing to Chronic Sympathetic Activation

(from Curtis and O'Keefe, Mayo Clinical Proceedings, 2002)

Medical Conditions
Congestive heart failure
Depression, anxiety
Hypertension
Insulin resistance or diabetes
Obesity
Sleep apnea

Psychosocial and Behavioral Conditions
Abuse of stimulants
Chronic stress
Hostility
Sedentary lifestyle
Sleep deprivation
Smoking
Social isolation
Unhealthy diet

---

pressure, a jolt of adrenaline, or in response to an icy cold stimulus. Spasm can even be triggered by going outside on a cold winter day and getting a sudden chill. An unfortunately increasing cause of coronary spasm is the recreational use of cocaine; this can lead to heart attacks in susceptible people.

Damage to the heart muscle. Those catecholamines that jolt the heart and brain during stress can actually be toxic to the cells in your heart muscle. They can weaken the muscle and cause changes in the electrical impulse conduction, which can worsen heart failure and can result in a serious arrhythmia. Prolonged exposure to catecholamines in the days and weeks after heart attack can further injure surviving myocardial cells around the infarcted, or damaged, area.

How Beta-Blockers Work

Because catecholamines alter the function of the skin, muscles, lungs, brain, and eyes, you may wonder how they communicate with so many different types of cells. The cells in these tissues have receptors, called beta-adrenergic receptors, that accept a message from one or more of these chemicals to do whatever these cells are programmed to do during stress. This may be to constrict, dilate, shut down, or mobilize, depending on the type of tissue. These beta-adrenergic receptors are broadly classed into alpha-type and beta-type receptors. Beta-blocking drugs are designed to preferentially compete with catecholamines that affect the beta-type receptors. Heart tissue is primarily equipped with beta receptors, so blocking these receptors with a beta-blocker keeps your heart from pounding furiously every time you feel stress.

Benefits of Beta-Blockers

Beta-blockers provide several critical benefits to your heart.

Decreased need for oxygen. By slowing the heart rate and tempering the contractions, a beta-blocker reduces the amount of oxygen your heart requires, in the same way that the muscles in your legs need less oxygen when you're walking than they do when you're running.

Increased oxygen supply. Flow in the coronary arteries occurs primarily during the relaxation phase (diastole) of the cardiac cycle. During the heart's contraction, the tightening muscle squeezes the coronary arteries and interrupts the flow of oxygen-rich blood to the heart muscle. As your heart rate slows, the pause in between beats lengthens, which increases the amount of blood that reaches the heart muscle. For example, without a beta-blocker, that blood supply might be interrupted 90 times per minute. With a beta-blocker, it will only have 60 interruptions per minute.

Improved pumping efficiency. When the heart races, it beats faster but it may fill and empty less efficiently in patients with heart disease. Maintaining a lower heart rate allows the ventricle to fill completely and pump at maximum efficiency.

Decreased myocardial wall stress. When you are under chronic stress, the heart is continually stimulated by the sympathetic nervous system so that the heart never really gets a chance to rest. This inability to rest can cause the ventricle to become weak and dilated over time, and can lead to heart failure. By reducing the pressure against which the heart contracts, beta-blockers can help reduce wall stress.

Decreased risk of arrhythmias. If you are recovering from a heart attack, you are especially vulnerable to arrhythmias. The electrical activity of the heart can become disorganized as impulses move around and through the area of ischemic heart muscle damage. If the impulses become disorganized to a sufficient extent, ventricular tachycardia or ventricular fibrillation can occur. If your sympathetic nervous system is working in high gear, and you have a rapid heart rate, you are at increased risk for serious arrhythmia. By contrast, reducing your heart rate, and reducing the nervous impulses and circulating chemicals of the sympathetic nervous system will reduce your potential for arrhythmia.

Reduced size of infarction. If you do have a heart attack, being on beta-blocking medication may reduce the amount of damage your heart muscle suffers as a result. Here's how it works. The sympathetic nervous system is the first part of your body to respond to any medical emergency. The pain and fear that accompany a heart attack will stress your heart at the moment when it has the least energy to spare. Blocking the beta receptors will limit additional stimulation to the heart and help protect the heart muscle by reducing its demand for oxygen while you seek medical attention.

Slowed atherosclerotic growth. By reducing blood pressure, beta-blockers may reduce the damage high blood pressure causes to the endothelial cells that line the blood vessel walls. Injury to the blood vessel walls encourage the build up of plaque and can lead to obstructive blood clot. Lowered blood pressure can also reduce the incidence of a small tear in an atherosclerotic plaque causing the plaque to become unstable.

Types of Beta-Blockers

There are two major types of beta-adrenergic receptors that can be affected by catecholamines, the chemicals released into the blood stream during stress.

Beta-1 receptors are found in the heart. Their job is to increase heart rate and the force of each heartbeat.

Beta-2 receptors are found in the smooth muscle cells in the airways and blood vessels of the lungs and when stimulated cause widening of the airway passages and lung blood vessels.

Beta-Blocker Selectivity

Beta-blocking drugs can selectively block the activity of specific types of beta-receptors.

Beta-1 selective. These drugs block the activity of beta-1 receptors, which are primarily located in cardiac muscle. This reduces your heart rate and decreases the contractile force of the heart. Because they don't affect the beta-2 receptors in the lungs and other organs, these drugs can modify cardiac function without the risk causing a tightening of the airways in people who have asthma.

Beta-selective. If a medication is beta-selective, that means that it blocks both beta-1 and beta-2 receptors, but leaves alpha receptors unaffected, including those that constrict blood vessels in the skin and extremities. Leaving these alpha receptors alone can occasionally cause some side effects for people with peripheral circulation problems, if the unblocked alpha receptors promote constriction of these arteries.

Unselective. These drugs block alpha and beta receptors alike and have the greatest ability to counteract the combined effects of all of the catecholamines. By blocking the alpha receptors, these drugs also help dilate the arteries. By doing so, these medications can lower blood pressure and improve circulation. Unselective beta-blockers are useful in treating hypertension, left ventricular dysfunction, and some forms of heart failure. However, in practice, the combined effect of an unselective beta-blocker is more often achieved by combining a beta-1 selective drug with an ACE inhibitor or another vasodilator.

Lipophilic vs. hydrophilic. Lipophilic beta-blockers bind more strongly to fatty cells, including those of the brain and the central nervous system. By crossing the blood brain barrier, they may more easily affect the stress response, but for the same reason, these agents may produce depression in some patients.

Who Should Take Beta-Blockers?

Beta-blockers have been used routinely to prevent secondary heart attacks and other coronary events for more than 20 years.

According to guidelines created by the American Heart Association/American College of Cardiology, most patients trying to prevent a second heart attack are good candidates for beta-blocker therapy, provided they don't have certain other medical conditions, such as serious asthma. Yet, these drugs are often underprescribed.

Your doctor may prescribe a beta-blocker for many reasons.

Help Prevent Another Heart Attack

Anyone recovering from a heart attack should be considered for beta-blocker therapy—unless there is a clear reason why someone should not be taking this medication. This is true even for individuals who needed primary angioplasty or clot-busting therapy while hospitalized. Patients who develop stable angina or who suffer from angina after bypass surgery should also be considered for beta-blockers as a means of protecting the heart from the effects of stress and exertion. A beta-blocker is an ideal tool to reduce the likelihood of further cardiac events, including sudden cardiac death among patients with complex ventricular arrhythmias.

Beta-blockers are such a standard therapy for treating acute myocardial infarction that this therapy often begins in the hospital and continues for the long term at home. In patients who tolerate the drugs well, beta-blocker therapy can continue indefinitely. There is no arbitrary age limit for the use of beta-blockers in patients with coronary artery disease. In fact, patients over the age of 60 can derive the greatest benefits from this drug.

Help Prevent Heart Failure

If you have suffered a severe myocardial infarction, particularly one that damaged a large portion of the anterior wall of the left ventricle, you may be at high risk for developing heart failure. During the healing process, this damaged area will not be able to pump blood. Instead, this portion of the muscle will stretch and thin over time. The area around the infarction will naturally thicken and strengthen to compensate for the part of the heart that's not working. If the ventricle can eventually make up for that damaged area that no longer functions, then the healing will lead to normal or near normal pumping function of the ventricle. If not, the heart muscle will continue to thicken and dilate, which can lead to heart failure.

Some of this recovery process takes place in the hospital, but it can continue for months afterward. Beta-blockers assist by reducing the amount of work the heart has to do as it heals.

If you have left ventricular (LV) dysfunction, your doctor may prescribe both a beta-blocker and an ACE inhibitor to more fully control your sympathetic nervous system and your blood pressure. An ACE inhibitor is a drug that lowers blood pressure by acting indirectly to relax resistance in the arteries.

In recent studies, patients with LV dysfunction who took both a beta-blocker and an ACE inhibitor had an increased survival rate compared to those patients taking either drug alone.

Slow the Progression of Heart Failure

Recent studies indicate that hyperactivity of the sympathetic nervous system encourages the progression of mild and moderate heart failure to severe heart failure. Therefore, a beta-blocker, used carefully and judiciously under the supervision of your doctor, can slow this process by keeping the heart from overtaxing itself in daily life.

Patients who suffer from heart failure are also at special risk for serious, and potentially fatal, ventricular arrhythmias.

Manage Stable Angina

Beta-blockers are very effective in treating effort-induced angina (also called stable angina) because they keep the heart from racing and pounding during physical and emotional stress. As a result, they reduce the heart's need for oxygen.

Beta-blocking drugs are often combined with nitrates, such as nitroglycerin, in the treatment of chronic angina. These medications increase the blood flow through obstructed coronary vessels, by relaxing and opening up the arteries. For the same reason, beta-blockers are also frequently combined with calcium antagonists, another medication that dilates arteries.

Lower Hypertension

Beta-blockers lower blood pressure and decrease the chance of heart attack and stroke in both younger and older adults with hypertension. These drugs also help prevent people with high blood pressure from developing left ventricular dysfunction as a result of their hypertension.

When I go in to do my stress test, they try to get my heart rate up and really get it going, but I'm on this beta-blocker so it doesn't really work. Jeff G.

Side Effects and Complications

Fortunately, there are few drug interaction issues with beta-blockers. However, there are other side effects and complications you should be aware of.

AV block. Patients who are predisposed to a type of irregular heart rhythm known as atrioventricular heart block may find that a beta-blocker aggravates this condition. This is because the drug slows the conduction of the signal from the atrium to the ventricle. However, it is quite unusual for patients with normal conduction tissue to develop heart block while on beta-blockers, and when necessary, pacemakers can be used to control heart rates that are too slow. Some calcium channel blockers, when combined with beta-blockers, can cause AV block.

Excessive bradycardia. In some people, beta-blockers can lower the heart rate to below safe levels. An abnormally low heart rate, called bradycardia, can lead to weakness, fainting, and sometimes to angina and heart failure.

Hypotension. A beta-blocker can reduce your blood pressure. If it drops too low, you may experience episodes of dizziness and light-headedness, especially when getting up from a seated or reclining position. It is often possible to reduce the dose or eliminate the use of another medication that is contributing to the problem of low blood pressure and continue the beta-blocker in the original or reduced dose.

Exercise. You may notice a decrease in your tolerance for exercise when you take beta-blockers. You may notice some slight dizziness when you increase your level of activity. These symptoms generally decrease with time. While it is true that competitive athletes often are aware of a decrease in physical capacity while taking beta-blockers, this is not generally true for patients who exercise to lower peak effort levels as part of a regular exercise program. As you will see, submaximal exercise tolerance is far more important to most cardiac patients than is maximal effort tolerance.

Quality of life. Beta-blockers have been reported to cause depression, fatigue, sexual dysfunction, and nightmares. These side effects make sense since the sympathetic nervous system helps elevate mood, wakefulness and sexual function. And yet, heart disease and heart surgery are such life changing events that they often trigger depression, fatigue, sexual dysfunction, and difficulty sleeping even in the absence of beta-blockers.

What the Research Shows

A group of researchers recently reviewed 15 studies to determine what percentage of people taking beta-blockers reported these side effects compared to those receiving placebo. The study found no statistically significant association between beta-blockers and depression. Further, they found that fatigue did affect more people on beta-blockers than on placebo, but this amounted to just one extra case of fatigue for every 57 patients taking the drugs.

As for the correlation between beta-blockers and sexual dysfunction, the researchers found that 21.6 percent of people taking beta-blockers reported sexual dysfunction, but then so did 17.4 percent of the people taking placebo. Although some cases of sexual dysfunction can be directly attributed to beta-blockers, many cannot.

Who Should Not Take Beta-Blockers

As important as beta-blockers are to the routine management of most forms of coronary artery disease, not everyone may require these drugs. The following conditions may affect the likelihood of your use of beta-blockers.

Low risk patients. If you have survived a mild heart attack, have no ventricular dysfunction, hypertension, or elevated heart rate, and have done well on your pre-discharge or outpatient exercise test, your doctor may not prescribe a beta-blocker. In your case, the chances that you will suffer short-term cardiovascular complications are relatively low so your doctor may not believe that you require chronic beta-blocker therapy. Also, if you have had undergone a successful bypass or angioplasty, your doctor may not believe that you need this drug.

Variant angina (due to coronary spasm). This is a fairly rare type of angina caused by a spasm in the coronary arteries that reduces blood flow to the heart. The condition is generally not related to exercise or to stress, but rather occurs during periods of relative rest. In rare patients with this type of angina, beta-blockers may not be appropriate because they sometimes can worsen the spasm.

Low heart rate. Beta-blockers slow the heart rate, and too much of the drug can slow the heart rate too much. If your heart rate at rest is already low, say below 60 beats per minute, or if there is evidence of slowed electrical activity within the heart, your doctor may be concerned that beta-blockers might not be right for you.

However, while your heart rate may well be relatively slow at rest, angina and ischemia generally occur during exercise or during stress when your heart rate is much higher. When this occurs, beta-blockers may be appropriate and useful, particularly in a moderate dose.

Signs of peripheral hypoperfusion. Hypoperfusion means that blood flow to the tissues is not adequate for normal function. Blocking the beta receptors while leaving the alpha receptors alone may cause trouble for some patients with poor circulation due to obstructive atherosclerosis in the peripheral arteries. Alpha activity causes most of the body's blood vessels to constrict, which will exacerbate this circulatory problem. It can even worsen hypertension in some cases.

Very low blood pressure. If your systolic pressure is very low at rest—under 90 mm Hg—beta-blockers may reduce your blood pressure to even lower levels, which can result in symptoms such as dizziness.

Beta-Blockers and Diabetes

People with diabetes know that an increased heart rate can be a signal of hypoglycemia. Obviously, keeping the heart rate artificially low can mask the signs of hypoglycemia. Also, the sympathetic nervous system has a minor role in helping to regulate blood sugar. When blood sugar levels fall too low, it is the sympathetic nervous system that urges the liver to release stored fat and make more glucose, or energy, available to the body. Using a beta-blocker to inhibit the effects of the sympathetic nervous system can reduce its natural and beneficial effect on the way your body processes and releases energy, and can therefore prolong episodes of hypoglycemia.

Even so, the benefits of beta-blockers in patients with diabetes is so clear that this caution should not prevent the use of these life-extending drugs. The incidence of reinfarction and sudden death following a heart attack for people with diabetes is much higher than for people who don't have the condition. Therefore the potential benefits of beta-blockers are especially strong in this population, and

---

An Important Warning

You should never stop beta-blocking medication on your own. This is an important warning that cannot be overstated. An abrupt withdrawal can have severe consequences. The sudden rebound activation of the sympathetic nervous system can exacerbate angina or bring on another heart attack. If you suffer from hypertension, the sudden increase in blood pressure can cause angina, rapid heart beat, anxiety, or perspiration. People at high risk for another heart attack are particularly vulnerable to the negative effects of withdrawal. Those who stop their beta-blockers abruptly and without supervision are at risk for consequences that include unstable angina, heart attack, and sudden death from arrhythmia. If you do need to discontinue using one of these drugs, your doctor can supervise a regimen in which you reduce the dosage safely over the course of several weeks.

---

most doctors now routinely use beta-blockers despite diabetes in patients with coronary disease. Also, hypoglycemia occurs less often when taking cardioselective beta-1 blockers.

Some Questions to Ask

By now you know that stress causes your sympathetic nervous system to push your heart into overdrive—a condition that can cheat your heart of oxygen it needs to function. If you are recovering from a heart attack, angioplasty or bypass surgery, or if you suffer from arrhythmia, your doctor may recommend that you take a beta-blocker to protect your heart against the effects of stress. Some questions you should think about and then ask your doctor are:

* *Is my lifestyle very stressful?*
* *Do I have a medical condition that could cause chronic sympathetic activation?*
* *Am I at high risk for a heart attack?*
* *If any of the above are true, am I a good candidate for beta-blocker therapy?*
* *What type of beta-blocker would be right for me?*
* *What side effects should I be aware of?*
* *How will beta-blockers affect my other medical conditions, including diabetes, circulatory problems, or kidney or liver disease?*
* *How long will I be on this medication?*

Chapter 8

◆ ◆ ❖ ◆ ◆ ◆ ❖ ◆ ◆ ❖ ◆ ◆ ◆ ❖ ◆ ◆ ❖ ◆ ◆

ACE Inhibitors and ARBs

Reducing Blood Pressure
and Improving Blood Flow

If you've had a heart attack or are at high risk for having one, your doctor may prescribe a medication called an angiotensin-converting enzyme (ACE) inhibitor or an angiotensin receptor blocker (ARB) to reduce your blood pressure and improve blood flow through your arteries.

In this chapter you'll learn how your kidneys help control your blood pressure using a substance called angiotensin, and why people with heart disease often have an excess of angiotensin in their systems. This excess can exacerbate many of the problems caused by heart disease, including angina, heart attacks, and heart failure. Blocking or reducing the effects of this substance can have important benefits to many people with heart disease. Before taking an ACE inhibitor or ARB, you will want to become familiar with common precautions and side effects, and you will want to learn how this medication will interact with others you may be taking.

Why Blood Pressure Matters

Decades ago, doctors thought it was important to raise the blood pressure of people suffering or recovering from acute myocardial infarction. Higher blood pressure was thought to stave off the symptoms of shock, a condition in which the body's systems shut down for lack of blood flow to the organs. It was then common practice to give a patient medication to constrict arteries throughout the body, artificially raising the patient's blood pressure for days after the heart attack.

We now know that the opposite is true. A heart already in trouble should not be further taxed by having to pump against constricted arteries, particularly if those arteries have already been narrowed by atherosclerosis. Constriction of the major arteries makes it more difficult for your heart to pump blood, which actually reduces blood flow to the organs and tissues of your body. Also, the harder your heart has to work, the more oxygen it needs, but in the presence of heart disease and constricted arteries, that oxygen supply may be limited. As a result, the heart weakens further, which may lead to heart failure.

In contrast, dilating the arteries lowers the force opposing the heart muscle as it pumps blood. This lowered resistance can actually increase blood flow from the weakened heart and can help keep your blood pressure stable at safe levels.

Blood Pressure In Recovery

Increasing blood flow to coronary arteries is crucial during a heart attack. Even as myocardial cells in one section of the heart are dying because of an acute blockage, the heart muscle is still working to contract with each heartbeat. Trying to pump blood into resistant arteries costs the heart much more energy, which means that myocardial cells will die at a much faster rate. Preventing this situation is a priority for you if you are at high risk for suffering a heart attack, or if you are currently recovering from one. In these conditions, your doctor is likely to prescribe an angiotensin converting enzyme (ACE) inhibitor or an angiotensin receptor blocker (ARB). These drugs help control your blood pressure by allowing your arteries to relax or dilate when they need to. In turn, this increases the pumping efficiency of the heart while reducing its workload.

An ACE inhibitor is particularly important if you are recovering from a heart attack in which your left ventricle suffered large areas of damage. This drug is also useful if you have symptoms of heart

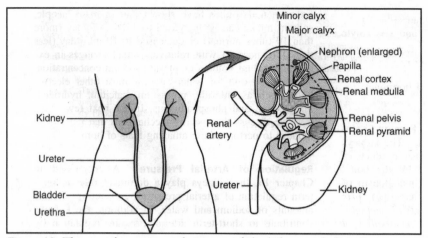

Figure 10: The general anatomy and structure of the kidneys and the urinary system. Within each kidney, blood from the renal artery is filtered to regulate salt and water balance and to excrete waste products in the urine.

failure or have diabetes, even if you did not suffer from high blood pressure prior to your heart attack or surgery. These conditions make you more sensitive to the harmful effects of a substance in the blood called angiotensin, which increases resistance to blood flow and raises pressure in the arteries throughout your body.

How Your Body Controls Blood Pressure

Your body's blood pressure is fine-tuned throughout the day by your renal-adrenal system, which includes the kidneys and the adrenal glands (see Figure 10). Its primary task is to prevent blood pressure from falling to dangerously low levels. This system increases blood pressure in a couple of ways. It controls the amount of fluid in the body, extracting water and sodium from the blood when there is too much fluid, triggering retention of salt and water and thirst when there is too little. In general, blood pressure can increase and decrease in direct relation to the volume of fluid in the body.

The kidneys also possess a method for rapidly increasing blood pressure in times of crisis by constricting arteries to raise resistance (and also veins to increase the volume of blood in the central circulation) throughout the body. They have to be able to do this, because although the kidneys make up just 0.4 percent of your body weight, they require about 22 percent of the heart's output of blood in order to function. Therefore, they are acutely sensitive to any reduction in blood flow.

For example, if you were to suffer an injury that caused you to hemorrhage blood, the renal system would sense the resulting drop in blood pressure and blood flow and take steps to preserve fluid and constrict the arteries in order to maintain blood pressure and circulation to the vital organs. This would help keep you alive.

When blood pressure or blood supply to the kidneys drops for any reason, the kidneys release a hormone called renin into the blood stream. As renin circulates, it acts on a protein in the blood called angiotensinogen, which it breaks down into a simpler substance, called a protein peptide—angiotensin I. When this peptide encounters a chemical in the body called angiotensin-converting enzyme (ACE), it is further transformed into angiotensin II, a substance that significantly alters your circulation.

What Angiotensin Does

Angtiotensin II has a number of effects on the body (see Figure 11):

It constricts arteries. Arteries contain smooth muscle cells that allow them to dilate and constrict as they need to in order to move blood. Angiotensin II binds with receptors inside these cells throughout the body causing the arteries to constrict and rapidly raise blood pressure.

It constricts veins. Ordinarily, veins are loose reservoirs of relatively slow-moving blood. In the presence of angiotensin II, they push more blood back to the heart and increase the body's blood volume, and therefore, its blood pressure

It traps blood in the kidneys. This enables the kidneys to better filter out impurities.

It increases blood volume. Angiotensin II stimulates thirst. It also promotes water and sodium retention in the body. Getting salt and water into the system and keeping it there is another way to raise

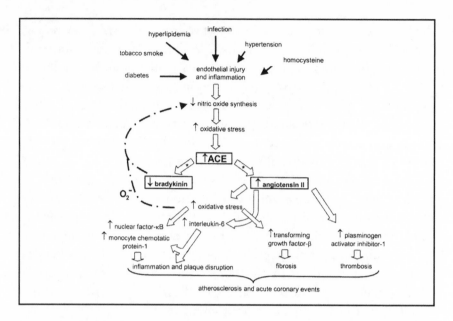

Figure 11: The role of tissue angiotensin-converting enzyme (ACE) and angiotensin II in the complex inflammatory reactions underlying atherosclerosis and acute coronary syndromes.

blood pressure and to protect fluid volume over the course of several hours and days.

All of this is quite normal. When your blood pressure is in danger of falling too low, the renin-angiotensin system helps your kidneys raise your body's blood volume and pressure to normal levels. Quite often, however, a chronic disorder, such as coronary artery disease, or a sudden trauma, such as a heart attack, overstimulates this system. This can complicate your recovery from surgery or from a heart attack. Angiotensin is a great asset for regulation of body fluid volume and blood pressure under normal and under most stress situations. But in heart disease, angiotensin is a danger.

How Angiotensin Builds Up in Your System

The renin-angiotensin system is activated whenever there is a drop in arterial blood flow to the kidneys. This decrease could be caused by any of a number of occurrences including:

* *Severe hemorrhage*
* *Partial blockage of renal arteries due to atherosclerosis*
* *Weakness of the heart following a heart attack*
* *Poor pumping ability by the left ventrical*
* *Heart failure*

When you are having a heart attack, or even when you suffer an episode of angina, the stress and pain you feel will also stimulate the sympathetic nervous system and trigger the renin–angiotensin system.

The renin–angiotensin system works well when your heart is healthy, but not so well when your heart muscle is ailing because of coronary trauma or because your arteries have been narrowed significantly by plaque. If you have had a heart attack, or if you have frequent episodes of angina, there is a significant possibility that there is also too much angiotensin already circulating in your system, keeping your arteries taught and narrow, and further complicating your heart disease. Merely having arterial plaque can affect the way your arteries respond to the angiotensin in your blood. Atherosclerosis changes the cells in your arteries, making them more sensitive to angiotensin, while making them less sensitive to competing chemicals that can dilate the arteries, and improve blood flow to your heart and other organs.

Blocking Angiotensin

There are two ways to block the effects of angiotensin on the circulatory system. The first is to interrupt the chain of chemical events that leads to the transformation of angiotensin I into angiotensin II. This is done by a drug called an ACE inhibitor. It limits the function of angiotensin converting enzyme, the chemical that enables that transformation.

The second method is to block the receptors in the arteries that react to angiotensin. A newer type of drugs, called angiotensin receptor blockers (ARB), does just that. Although more research has been done on the older ACE inhibitor class of drugs, initial studies suggest that the newer angiotensin receptor blockers are likely to have comparable value in the management of coronary artery disease.

Angiotensin receptor blockers are a more selective way to block the renin-angiotensin system, because they block the effects of the chemical rather than limiting or preventing its formation. ARBs produce a slightly different effect in the system than ACE inhibitors, which act by reducing the amount of angiotensin that is circulating in your body.

Inhibitors Versus Blockers

The differences between the two drugs may seem trivial, but they aren't. A major difference between ACE inhibitors and ARBs is that ACE inhibitors also modify other chemicals in your body that also depend on the angiotensin-converting enzyme. One of these is bradykinin, a chemical that has a powerful relaxation effect on the arteries. ACE breaks down bradykinin in the arteries. Therefore, inhibition of ACE in your system may increase the amount of bradykinin, which makes your arteries more likely to dilate when they need to. Some researchers think that this is an important advantage of ACE inhibitors over the newer ARBs.

On the other hand, one of the annoying and sometimes limiting side effects of ACE inhibitors is a persistent, and otherwise unexplained cough. It seems that this cough is caused, at least in part, by an increase of bradykinin in the lungs. This side effect is not present with ARBs.

So far, the published research on the effectiveness of ARBs in patients after a heart attack are not as established as the data for ACE inhibitors. Because ARBs are a newer class of drug, there have been few head-to-head comparisons with ACE inhibitors and little published research on the ARB's long-term effects on heart disease. ARBs do seem very effective for the treatment of high blood pressure and for reducing the hypertrophy, or dilation, of the left ventricle that is such a threat to people with heart muscle damage or a long history of high blood pressure. ARBs may prove to be as beneficial as ACE inhibitors in ischemic disease, and may become a standard treatment for secondary prevention in the future, but more research is required to definitively establish this.

Benefits of Reducing Angiotensin

Reduced infarction size. If you have had a myocardial infarction, you were probably given an ACE inhibitor or an ARB in the hospital to help lower arterial resistance in an effort to ease the workload of the heart and reduce the size of the infarction. The stress and pain of a heart attack activates the renin-angiotensin system and begins to increase the resistance of your arteries. In the hours following a heart attack, some of the cells in the infarcted area die, while others lie dormant until the healing process begins. If the workload of the heart is increased at this time, the dormant cells that would otherwise heal will die instead. Lowering the level of angiotensin in your system reduces the stress on those dormant cells, which may allow them to survive.

Reduced scarring. Angiotensin released in the heart promotes the production of scar tissue in the injured heart muscle after a heart attack. This is a normal and desirable part of the healing process. If the damaged area is small, the dead tissue scars over while the surrounding tissue tries to recover. If, on the other hand, there is a large area of damage on the heart muscle, the rapid development of scar tissue encouraged by angiotensin becomes a problem. As this damaged area scars over, it becomes stiff and noncompliant. This stiffness can limit the ability of the ventricle to fill normally with blood during its relaxation phase. Large amounts of scar can cause the heart muscle around the injured area to work harder to contract. These problems can lead to heart failure.

Reduced ventricular remodeling. In the healing process that follows a heart attack, the dead cells in the infarcted area scar over, while the injured but dormant cells surrounding that area either die or revive. All this time, the healthy tissue around the infarction is carrying on with its business of contracting and relaxing to move blood in and out of the ventricle without any help from the infarcted area. In its attempt to compensate for the damaged area, the healthy heart muscle grows thicker and stronger—a process called ventricular remodeling. If the stronger heart muscle still can't adapt, the stress of trying to pump blood will cause the ventricle to dilate. As the ventricle enlarges, it becomes even less able to pump blood efficiently. If it continues to dilate, the heart will eventually fail to pump enough blood to meet the demands of the tissues throughout the body.

By reducing resistance in the arteries and improving blood flow, and by slowing the process of scarring, an ACE inhibitor or ARB can actually reduce the amount of abnormal ventricular remodeling that the heart endures in the healing process.

Reduced likelihood of heart failure. If you have been diagnosed with left ventricular (LV) dysfunction, it means that your heart's main pumping chamber (the left ventricle) isn't pumping blood as it should. Your doctor will probably talk to you about your heart's ejection fraction. With each heartbeat a healthy ventricle will pump out 50 to 60 percent or more of the blood it contains. As the heart is damaged by the scarring of infarction or impeded in contraction by high arterial resistance, the ejection fraction can decrease to 40 percent or below. Ejection fractions below 30 percent after a heart attack are common. If the heart mends itself well, the ejection fraction can increase again, and progression toward heart failure can stop. If not, some degree of heart failure is likely.

Taking an ACE inhibitor or ARB can be crucial to patients who have left ventricular dysfunction but do not have heart failure, because these drugs increase the effectiveness of each heartbeat. By dilating arteries and arterioles, an ACE inhibitor or ARB reduces the resistance the blood encounters when it leaves the heart after each contraction. This increases the blood flow to the organs and tissues of the body. The lowered resistance can provide a real boost to the circulatory system. Just by getting blood to the capillaries, an ACE inhibitor or ARB can slow the progress of heart failure and improve the way you feel. It can also reduce the likelihood of complications from ventricular dysfunction, including chest pain, shortness of breath, swelling of the legs, arrhythmias, heart attack, and hospitalization.

Improved symptoms of heart failure. If you have left ventricular failure, taking an ACE inhibitor or ARB can reduce your symptoms.

As your circulation improves, you will be less likely to suffer from shortness of breath, difficulty breathing while lying down, and general fatigue. As your heart begins to function better, you will have less of a tendency to retain the salt and water that cause swelling in the legs. Better cardiac function will also help reduce the buildup of fluid in the lungs that causes shortness of breath in heart failure. These changes may reduce the amount of diuretic medication you need to maintain a normal fluid balance in your body.

What the Research Shows

The Heart Outcomes Prevention Evaluation (HOPE) trial was designed as a long-term evaluation of a wide range of heart patients to see if ACE inhibition would help prevent another heart attack or coronary event. The benefit was so clear—a 22 percent reduction in heart attack, stroke and death in patients treated with ACE inhibition—that the study was halted prematurely.

In the Studies of Left Ventricular Dysfunction trial (SOLVD), researchers found that the treatment with this class of drugs produced a 26 percent reduction in death and heart failure serious enough to require repeat hospitalization. In another study, patients who took ACE inhibitors had a 25 percent reduced rate of recurrent myocardial infarction compared to patients taking placebo.

Even people with the most severe degree of heart failure can notice significant improvement in these areas. One study noted that more than 40 percent of class IV patients (defined as those patients with symptoms even at rest) taking ACE inhibitors improved their heart function and had higher survival rates at the end of the two-year study. These findings, and many others, have demonstrated that taking an ACE inhibitor dramatically improves survival and quality of life for people suffering from heart failure.

Reduced likelihood of another heart attack. Several studies have shown that ACE inhibitors benefit a broader range of patients with coronary disease than only those suffering from LV dysfunction or heart failure, and that these drugs have benefits beyond reducing arterial resistance and improving circulation. There is a growing body of evidence that suggests that angiotensin plays a role in creating and eventually destabilizing arterial plaque. If that is so, then reducing angiotensin should delay the progress of coronary artery disease and prevent future heart attacks.

Who Should Take ACE Inhibitors or ARBs

According to current American Heart Association/American College of Cardiology guidelines, anyone who has suffered a heart attack should be treated with an ACE inhibitor indefinitely.

However, since all general guidelines have exceptions, your doctor may decide that this recommendation is not appropriate for your situation. If you have no complications during your recovery from a heart attack, and specifically if you have no evidence of left ventricular dysfunction, your doctor may decide that you no longer need an ACE inhibitor or ARB after a month or two. That's because there's still no evidence that people with the lowest risk of having another heart attack or coronary event will definitely benefit from long-term medication to reduce angiotensin in the system.

Those at lowest risk include:

* *People under the age of 65 who have suffered a small amount of damage during their heart attacks or who have suffered no significant damage of the left ventricle.*

* *People whose ejection fraction, the amount of blood pumped out of the ventricle with each heart beat, is greater than 50 percent (which is considered near normal).*

Research to support long-term ACE inhibition or use of ARBs even among lowest risk patients could come along at any time. Even in the absence of this conclusive research, some cardiologists feel that the beneficial effects of ACE inhibitors on the arteries make them an important preventative measure for all patients with atherosclerosis.

People with Diabetes

If you have diabetes, you are at increased risk of both coronary artery disease and renal disease. For you, an ACE inhibitor or ARB is a particularly important tool in fighting the effects of atherosclerotic disease.

At least one study of ACE inhibitors, the HOPE study, included a significant number of people with diabetes who had survived a heart attack. The ACE inhibitor delayed or prevented coronary events in these individuals, particularly subjects with hypertension and a low ejection fraction. The people who took the ACE inhibitor also showed a significant reduction in diabetic complications.

Dosing

As beneficial as ACE inhibitors and ARBs can be, dosing is a delicate matter. Your doctor will probably begin with a low dose and increase gradually to avoid the major side effect of the drug, which is low blood pressure. It's important to take the medication exactly as it is prescribed to help the doctor arrive at a dosing that is optimal for you.

Precautions

Renal failure. Doctors are usually cautious about prescribing an ACE inhibitor or ARB to patients who have kidney failure, or blockages in both renal arteries. If you have this condition, the decision to take an ACE inhibitor is a risk-benefit issue that you need to discuss with your doctor. If you do take an ACE inhibitor or ARB, it is important that your kidney function be monitored carefully.

Low blood pressure. An ACE inhibitor or ARB might not be well tolerated by patients whose systolic blood pressure is below 100 mm Hg, because it may further lower blood pressure and lead to symptoms such as dizziness. Blood pressure that is too low will ultimately decrease blood flow to vital organs.

Allergies. Some people are allergic to ACE inhibitors. If you have had an allergic reaction to this type of drug in the past, you should not be given one. In this situation, the angiotensin receptor blocking drugs (ARB) provide a useful alternative.

Pregnancy. Women who are pregnant should not take an ACE inhibitor or ARB because it might damage the developing fetus.

Side Effects

ACE inhibitors and ARBs are well tolerated by most patients, and most side effects that do occur can be reversed by stopping the medication.

The most common side effect is low blood pressure, particularly the first time you take it. This is generally not too much of a problem and may not recur with subsequent doses. But for this reason, your doctor may begin with a low starting dose and then increase the amount you take over time. Other side effects include dizziness, headaches, or mild azotemia, which is an accumulation of waste products in the blood due to decreased kidney function. Other people may experience itching or a rash; blood changes such as a build-up of potassium, a decrease in white blood cells or red blood cells, or an increase in blood platelets; or excess protein in the urine. Angioedema, a condition in which patches of skin swell and become infected, is a rare allergic reaction to this drug that prevents its future use.

One side effect of ACE inhibitors that many patients notice is a cough, which is perhaps caused by the increased effect of bradykinin in the lungs. It is annoying but not serious. If the cough becomes too uncomfortable, your doctor may switch you to another ACE inhibitor, or more likely to an angiotensin receptor blocker (ARB). Patients should be aware, though, that a worsening cough may be a symptom of heart failure and not a reaction to this drug.

Drug Interactions

Beta-blockers. If you are already taking a beta-blocking drug for secondary prevention of ischemic heart disease, addition of an ACE inhibitor or ARB may be advantageous. Activation of the sympathetic nervous system is one of the conditions that accelerates the development of heart failure. The beta-blocker will reduce your heart rate and the force of your heart's contractions, while the ACE inhibitor will reduce the resistance to blood flow in your arteries, among its other stabilizing effects on the arteries themselves. The people who will benefit most from this combination of drugs are those who are at highest risk. This includes patients who have severely reduced left ventricular function, measured by an ejection fraction less than 30 percent, or those who have kidney trouble. In this high-risk group, some studies estimate that one life can be saved for every five people treated with both drugs.

Aspirin. Data from the Studies of Left Ventricular Dysfunction (SOLVD) trials initially indicated that taking aspirin might decrease the effectiveness of ACE inhibitors, or that a combination of the two drugs might impair the function of the kidneys. But a larger review of available studies has shown that aspirin and ACE together combined to lower death rate, hospitalization, and other complications.

Antacids. These medications reduce the ability of ACE inhibitors to be absorbed through the stomach thereby reducing their therapeutic effects.

Diuretics. By lowering salt, water, and blood volume in the body, these drugs lower blood pressure. Adding an ACE inhibitor or ARB into the mix can magnify this effect by lowering arterial resistance. The combination of the two can sometimes lower blood pressure too much. To prevent this, your doctor will want to be sure that you are not too dehydrated from your diuretic when you start taking an ACE inhibitor or an ARB. Your doctor will do this with a simple clinical evaluation of your blood pressure, heart rate, venous pressure in the neck veins, and skin tissue.

Some Questions to Ask

If you are recovering from a heart attack, emergency angioplasty, or bypass surgery, you may already be taking an ACE inhibitor or angiotensin receptor blocker (ARB) in the months after your hospitalization. This is particularly true if you've suffered a heart attack that has significantly damaged the left, or anterior, ventricle of your heart. If you have high blood pressure, you may also already be taking one of these medications. Even if you are not currently taking an ACE inhibitor or ARB, it may be useful for you to have a discussion with your doctor about this medication and whether or not it is appropriate for you. Some questions you might ask are:

* *Am I taking an ACE inhibitor or ARB, and if so, why?*

* *How long will I be on this medication?*

* *What are the short-term and long-term benefits of this medication?*

* *What are the risks for me?*

* *What are the potential side effects or complications that I should be aware of?*

* *What blood tests will I be taking to make sure the medication is safe for me? How often will they be necessary?*

* *If I am not taking this medication, why not?*

Chapter 9

◆ ◆ ❖ ◆ ◆ ❖ ◆ ◆ ❖ ◆ ◆ ❖ ◆ ◆ ❖ ◆ ◆ ❖ ◆ ◆

Statins and Other Lipid-Lowering Medications
Combatting Atherosclerosis

Numerous studies have shown that lowering the amount of cholesterol in your blood will slow the progression of atherosclerosis and will reduce your changes of having a heart attack or developing unstable angina.

Most people who have heart disease need to dramatically improve their cholesterol profile, and the fastest way to achieve this dramatic change is through medication. In this chapter, you'll learn about cholesterol and why its rapid reduction is such a priority in the secondary prevention of heart disease. You'll also learn about statins and other medications to lower cholesterol, how they work, and how much they can improve your cholesterol levels.

The Body Needs Cholesterol

Although most digested fats become fuel for the body, cholesterol is a structural fat, meaning that it is reserved for certain crucial functions. For example, the body requires cholesterol to build and maintain the membranes of individual cells. Cholesterol is used in much greater quantities by the skin as a protective, waterproofing agent. It helps to form cholic acid in the liver, which in turn creates bile salts that promote digestion. It's also a building block for some the body's hormones including testosterone, progesterone, and estrogen.

Dietary fats and cholesterol are absorbed from the intestines and go directly to the liver, where they are processed. From there, these fats are packed up in molecules of various sizes, called lipoproteins, and sent into the blood stream so that they can be used by the tissues and organs of the body. This is where cholesterol can cause trouble for the cardiovascular system.

Types of Lipoproteins

Lipoproteins entering the blood stream begin as large particles known as very low density lipoproteins (VLDL). These consist primarily of triglycerides—dietary fats that will be used as energy. As the VLDL molecules break down into smaller intermediate density lipoprotiens (IDL), the triglyceride particles travel to fatty tissue where they are stored for later use. These IDL further break down into low density lipoproteins (LDL), which contain cholesterol headed for the tissues. After a tissue cell picks up an LDL particle and uses some of it, the leftover cholesterol joins with high density lipoproteins (HDL), which returns them to the liver for elimination as waste

Therefore, LDL brings cholesterol to the tissues of the body, while HDL removes it from the tissues of the body. For this reason, LDL cholesterol has become known as the "bad" cholesterol, while HDL has become known as the "good" cholesterol.

There is another form of lipoprotein that is released by the liver that is related to LDL called lipoprotein (a), which is pronounced as lipoprotein "little a." Lipoprotein (a) appears to be avidly attracted to developing atherosclerotic plaques, and it may turn out to be a risk factor of even greater importance than LDL in some susceptible people.

How Cholesterol Builds Plaque

There are several theories about how atherosclerotic plaque forms in the arteries, as discussed in Chapter 4. In each of these theories, the LDL particles play a primary role in creating or encouraging plaque to form. Whatever the main inciting cause, LDL in the inner arterial wall is a critical component of the buildup of plaque in the arteries. Over time, fatty deposits on the endothelial wall provoke an inflammatory type response. Lipid–laden macrophages become "foam cells" and produce a swelling and scarring response in the endothelium (inner lining of the artery). With more LDL cholesterol and further inflammation, these swellings become atherosclerotic plaque that grows over the years. This response can cause smooth muscle cells from the outer parts of the artery to invade the endothelium to produce further plaque enlargement and scarring. Plaque is therefore made up of both fatty and scar type material, often as a fat rich center topped by a fibrous cap. Plaques that are full of fatty deposits, as opposed to fibrous (scar-type) elements, are especially problematic. These unstable, lipoprotein-rich plaques seem to be more prone to rupture, which leads to platelet activation and to the thrombosis that causes complete blockage of blood flow in an artery. This, in turn, leads to heart attack or stroke.

Your Lipid Panel

You may be familiar with the blood tests that measure lipid levels. The findings of this blood test are reported as: Total Cholesterol, HDL, LDL, Triglycerides, and the Ratio of LDL to HDL.

Your target levels of cholesterol are going to change as your risk for having a heart attack or other complication from heart disease change. For example:

* *A person with no symptoms of heart disease and no cardiac risk factors could have a total cholesterol level as high as 239 mg/dL, with an LDL level as high as 159 mg/dL before his or her doctor might prescribe a cholesterol-lowering diet or suggest a drug regimen.*

* *Someone who has a couple of risk factors for heart disease, and whose total 10-year risk for having a heart attack is less than 20 percent, should probably have a total cholesterol number that's under 200 mg/dL with the LDL level under 130 mg/dL. Doctors are likely to suggest dietary changes to lower cholesterol levels to these numbers before initiating drug therapy unless the cholesterol levels are excessively high.*

How Low Is Low Enough For You?

People with heart disease who have a very high risk of suffering another event or needing a revascularization procedure have a far lower target cholesterol level because they have the most to gain from immediately removing cholesterol particles from the bloodstream. If you are a heart patient with an LDL level above 100 mg/dL, your doctor will probably prescribe a strict diet that is low in cholesterol and saturated fats. If your LDL level is above 130 mg/dl, you will need to start taking medications to reduce your LDL level to below 100 as quickly as possible. More recent research has suggested that lowering LDL to below 80 may provide further protection. Even with dietary changes, most people with coronary artery disease need drug therapy to lower their cholesterol levels, particularly as lower goals for LDL cholesterol become recommended for reducing risk of heart attack.

Cholesterol Goals for Secondary Prevention

These are the currently acceptable levels of cholesterol:

Total cholesterol	Less than 180 mg/dl
LDL	Less than 100 (ideally less than 80)
HDL	Greater than 45
Triglycerides	Less than 150
Ratio of LDL to HDL	Ideally less than 2

As researchers discover more about the effects of cholesterol on the circulatory system, they will continue to modify the levels of cholesterol that are acceptable, probably lowering them over time.

More aggressive guidelines backed by some preventive cardiologists and nutritionists recommend that all people lower their LDL levels to below 100 mg/dL. Does this mean that everyone, regardless of health status, should be on a strict diet or take cholesterol-lowering medication? Some people think this may be desirable, and large studies are underway to clarify the risks and benefits of such an approach to public health. This argument is an important one, but if you already have cardiovascular disease, the answer is clear: You need to be sure that your lipid levels are under control.

When Should You Be Tested?

Experts know that LDL cholesterol levels decline in the hours immediately following a coronary event. By the second day after a coronary procedure or heart attack, the LDL levels are at an artificially low level and may remain low for several weeks, only to increase once the healing process has begun. Therefore, it is important for you to have your cholesterol checked periodically after you recover from any cardiac event, because it might be higher during routine activities than it was while you were in the hospital.

If you have a very high LDL level, your doctor will probably conduct additional tests to rule out other causes for this condition. These would include undiagnosed diabetes, hypothyroidism, obstructive liver disease, and chronic renal failure.

Benefits of Lower Cholesterol

For nearly 20 years, studies have demonstrated the link between sharply lowering cholesterol and preventing a second or subsequent coronary event.

Studies have also shown that a lowered cholesterol level can significantly improve survival rates in the first 30 days after a heart attack, particularly if the lower level is maintained for six months. A high cholesterol level at discharge, on the other hand, sets the stage for another, potentially fatal, heart attack.

Since drugs lower cholesterol relatively slowly, and because these drugs can not immediately reduce the size of arterial plaque, how

---

What the Research Shows

The first major study to confirm the benefits of lowering choles-terol was the 1986 Scandinavian Simvastatin Survival Study, often called 4S. In this study, 4444 patients with angina or previous heart attack were given either a statin to reduce their serum cholesterol level or a placebo, and then followed for more than five years. The total cholesterol readings for the treatment group decreased by an average of 25 percent, while LDL levels decreased by 35 percent. There was a corresponding 42-percent reduction of risk in coronary death, and a 37-percent reduction in the risk of having a revascular-ization. These results were similar for those who began with moderately elevated cholesterol readings and for those who began with very high readings.

---

can they affect short-term survival after a heart attack? The answer to this is not completely known, but it appears that these drugs pro-vide some immediate stabilizing effect on coronary artery plaques. This is yet another reason for the widespread use of these drugs.

Reduced Arterial Plaque

Some arterial blockages are thick with smooth muscle cells and fibrous (scar) tissue, while others consist mainly of LDL particles in the form of fatty deposits. This latter group is the type of plaque that is most likely to rupture and cause a coronary event such as throm-bosis or stroke. These unstable, fatty deposits are the most dangerous type of blockages, but they also respond most favorably to dietary changes and lipid-lowering medications. They may actually regress as the levels of lipids decreases in the blood. A very low level of choles-terol in your blood, achieved through diet or drug therapy, will stabilize the plaque and reduce the number of new lesions along arterial walls.

Improved Arterial Flow

Lowering your level of LDL can improve the function of endothe-lial cells that line the arteries by reducing oxidized LDL particles that

---

What the Research Shows

In some studies, people who have had an angiogram to measure their arterial blockages, and then another angiogram after lowering their cholesterol, have shown less progression in their atherosclerotic plaque than those whose cholesterol levels have remained the same. A recent study using a high dose of a lipid-lowering drug suggested that reduction of LDL levels to the range of 70 to 80 might actually halt the progression of coronary disease. Less cholesterol in the system and higher levels of HDL cholesterol may therefore combine to reduce plaque fat, which makes the lesions more stable and less likely to rupture.

---

can irritate them. When the endothelial cells are able to function normally, they are better able to produce chemicals such as nitric oxide, which allows arteries to dilate when they need to improve blood flow.

I take cholesterol medication ever since I got my stent. I've got no problems with weight. I'm not the most healthy eater, but my cholesterol isn't that high. My doctor thinks that the medication will help me anyway, and I take it because it's not going to do any harm.
Oscar M.

I didn't have high cholesterol, but my doctor thought he could improve the ratio of HDL to LDL and he likes the secondary benefits of this cholesterol drug for people who've had cardiac events, so I take it.
Samuel S.

People with Diabetes

Diabetes also adds additional dimension to the dangers of high cholesterol. High levels of glucose in the blood seem to increase the uptake of LDL by tissues, which in turn may accelerate atherosclerosis. In addition, high levels of insulin promote production of cholesterol within cells of the body. People with insulin resistant diabetes (Type 2 diabetes) who have high blood sugar levels as well as high levels of insulin in the blood will have higher cholesterol levels in their blood because the cells are already making as much cholesterol as they need. Recent evidence has further suggested that high insulin levels in Type 2 diabetes (and in the metabolic syndrome) can accelerate the oxidation of LDL within cells.

When you lower your insulin levels by reducing your carbohydrate intake, your cells produce less cholesterol and begin to take more from the blood. The LDL particles are less likely to oxidize and your blood cholesterol levels go down. Keeping a tight control on blood sugar and insulin levels will help lower cholesterol and reduce the likelihood of developing heart disease.

How Low Is Enough?

Many studies have confirmed that significantly lowering LDL levels reduces every negative outcome of coronary artery disease—mortality, major nonfatal heart attacks, revascularizations, episodes of angina and strokes. This holds true even for people whose current cholesterol levels aren't very high.

What the Research Shows

One study looked at patients who had survived a heart attack and who had mean total cholesterol levels of 209 mg/dL and mean LDL levels of 139 mg/dL. Both of these readings are considered average. When these patients lowered their LDL levels to 100 mg/dL they had better survival rates. However, the cholesterol-lowering medication had a less dramatic effect on patients with starting LDL levels below 125 mg/dL.

Still other studies indicate that there may be no threshold for lowering lipids among people who are at extremely high risk for having another heart attack. For these people, achieving an LDL level below 80 mg/dL significantly reduces their risk of having another heart attack or needing revascularization. But some of this result may be caused by secondary effects of the medication itself, such as stabilizing plaques or improving endothelial function, which helps the arteries to dilate when they need to.

Cholesterol Levels After Surgery

If you are recovering from bypass surgery, your cholesterol levels are especially critical. The main hazard for bypass grafts is that the new vessels will become blocked by the same atherosclerosis that affected the original arteries. In the first year following your bypass, the grafted vessels may become occluded because of factors unrelated to your cholesterol levels. These include technical problems with the surgery, build-up of scar tissue, or clot formation. After that first year, your cholesterol level, particularly the LDL level, is the major culprit in causing occlusion.

Unfortunately, new bypass vessels can become clogged within a few years, even though the atherosclerosis in the surrounding arteries took decades to accumulate. Vein grafts seem to be more likely to develop new blockages than do arterial grafts. Because these blockages grow so quickly, they are often unstable, which means they are more likely to rupture, causing blood clots and possibly a heart attack. Fast-growing blockages may also require another bypass.

Aggressive lowering of LDL levels to below 100 mg/dL, or maybe even further, can reduce this risk. This will require a strict diet and probably drug treatment as well.

What the Research Shows

In one study, patients who had undergone bypass surgery in the preceding one to eleven years, and who did lower their LDL cholesterol to below 100 mg/dL, had nearly 30 percent less progression of atherosclerotic blockages in their vein grafts after four to five years. The rate of revascularization in the treatment group was also down 29 percent after four years.

Cholesterol in People Over 75

The link between high cholesterol and the risk of coronary artery disease diminishes as you grow older in spite of the fact that your overall risk of heart disease continues to increase as you age. Although high cholesterol tends to cause fewer problems in people over the age of 75, reducing cholesterol to recommended levels is still beneficial to people up to age 75. In one study, patients as old as 82 lowered their risk of death from coronary disease by lowering their cholesterol levels with medication.

Medications to Lower Cholesterol

In the months after you come home from the hospital following your heart attack, bypass surgery, or angioplasty, one of your primary goals will be to lower your cholesterol levels. For many people, the surest way to do this is with medication, so your doctor will probably talk to you about taking one or more of the following drugs.

Statins

The introduction of hydroxymethylglutaryl coenzyme A (HMG-CoA) reductase inhibitors in 1987 represented a revolution in secondary prevention. This class of drugs, generally known as statins, dramatically lowers cholesterol levels. Statins have now been prescribed for more than 15 years and are the safest and most powerful drugs yet available for lowering cholesterol. Depending on the dose, a statin can decrease your LDLs by 18-55 percent, increase your HDLs by 5 to 15 percent, and decrease your triglycerides by 7 to 30 percent.

In numerous studies, statins have been shown to reduce heart attack, stroke, and the need for surgery by about 25 percent. In other studies, mortality rates among people taking the medication have declined by as much as 35 percent. These studies started with high-risk patients with high cholesterol levels and recent cardiac events, but now have been progressively extended to normal populations of younger people with what appears to be comparable protective effects.

How they work. Your liver needs the HMG-CoA reductase enzyme to produce cholesterol. Inhibiting this enzyme limits the cholesterol your liver can produce. So instead it begins to recycle dietary cholesterol that already is circulating in the blood stream.

However, statins do more than simply lower the cholesterol circulating in the system. Some studies suggest that they may block cholesterol from accumulating in the arterial walls. They may also prevent foam cells already in the arterial wall from attracting and accumulating new LDL particles. Preventing this accumulation potentially helps stabilize plaque and prevent ruptures that cause blood clots. Statins can also improve the functioning of the endothelial cells that line arteries and reduce inflammation inside the arteries. In short, this class of drugs appears to slow or even reverse the progress of the disease.

Several of these drugs, including lovastatin (Mevacor) and simvastatin (Zocor), are "inactive drugs," which means they need to be broken down and activated in the liver. Therefore, people with liver dysfunction might not fully benefit from them. Other drugs, including pravastatin (Pravachol), are already active when they are absorbed, so they do not have this limitation.

Side effects. The primary side effects of statins—muscle pain and elevated liver enzymes—occur in less than 1 percent of all patients taking them. Your doctor will regularly test your liver enzymes to determine if the statin is adversely affecting your system. Muscle pain or weakness is more common in patients taking the drugs in high doses or in combination with cyclosporine, niacin, or fibrates. It also occurs in patients who already have muscular disorders. Less common side effects include nausea, fatigue, headaches, changes in bowel function, and skin rashes. These effects are generally readily reversible by lowering the dose of the drug, or by stopping it, or by switching to another drug.

In extremely rare cases, statin use can cause rhabdomyolysis, a rare condition in which skeletal muscle cells break down and release toxins into the blood stream. This condition begins with muscle aches and inflammation, weakness, nausea, and vomiting, and it can be signaled by the passing of dark urine. If not treated, it can be fatal. If you think you are experiencing side effects, your doctor can perform tests to see if you need to stop taking the drug.

Who should not take statins. If you are pregnant or considering becoming pregnant, you should not take statins. If you do take one of these medications and then find yourself unexpectedly pregnant, you should stop taking the drug immediately and contact your doctor.

Because the drug may be activated in your liver, patients with active or chronic liver disease should not take it without a discussion of risks and benefits with their doctor.

Drug interactions. Certain drugs increase the risk of side effects, such as erythromycin-type antibiotics, niacin in high doses, the immunosuppressant cyclosporine, certain antifungal drugs, and HIV protease inhibitors.

If you take a hydrogen-blocking antacid such as cimetidine (Tagamet) or ranitidine (Zantac), or an antisecretory drug for acid reflux such as omeprazole (Prilosec), you should probably take these medications two hours after you take your statin to prevent their interfering with the statin's absorption into your system.

One statin, called Baycol, was recently taken off the market because 31 patients died of rhabdomyolysis. This condition is a possible side effect of any statin, particularly if it is taken as part of a combination therapy with niacin or fibrates, although even in these cases it has been extremely rare with the other statins. Any patient taking a statin who experiences severe muscle aches or passes dark urine should contact a doctor immediately.

Dosage and timing. Because much of the cholesterol production in the liver takes place while you sleep, your doctor may tell you to take your statin medication before going to bed. The dose of statins is highly variable from drug to drug. Your doctor will likely start with a low dose and increase the dose as needed to obtain your goal level of LDL cholesterol.

> *I started to have muscle cramps in 2001, and I noticed some blood on the toilet paper. I went to the doctor and he said, you've been on the same cholesterol drug for a long time, and maybe we should try a different one. I switched shortly thereafter. I asked, can cholesterol medication do that? And he said, "It's not likely, but you've been on the same one for a while, it won't hurt to switch." Then I went to a gastroenterologist who sent me to a urologist. He found elevated PSA levels. And now I'm on the prostate adventure. So, it wasn't the cholesterol medication at all.*
> *Tim S.*

Bile Acid Sequestrants

How they work. Bile acid sequestrants are resins that bind to bile acids in the small intestine. Examples include cholestyramine, cholestipol, and cholsevelam. This binding prevents the normal reabsorption of these bile acids, which causes the bile acids to become depleted. Because bile acids contain significant amounts of cholesterol, these resins lead to cholesterol wasting, which reduces the body level as the liver converts more cholesterol into needed bile acids to replace the loss. This type of drug can reduce LDLs by 15 to 30 percent, and raise HDLs by 3 to 5 percent. It either has no effect on triglycerides or actually raises them slightly. A resin is sometimes prescribed in combination with a statin. In combination, these drugs can lower LDL levels by more than 45 percent.

Who should take them? A resin is generally effective for people who can't take a statin or other medication that acts throughout the body. This includes women who wish to become pregnant and children who have inherited a condition that causes abnormally high cholesterol levels. Sometimes they are used together with statins, and a series of studies with different statins, have shown synergistic effects of combined therapy.

Side effects. This drug acts in the small intestines, so many of the side effects are also centered in the digestive system. Side effects include nausea, constipation, exacerbation of hemorrhoids, and bloating. A resin may also decrease the absorption of other drugs in the system including thyroxine, warfarin, digitalis, statins and fibrates.

Who should not take resins. People with liver or kidney disease or those who have triglyceride levels over 400 mg/dl are not good candidates for resins. Many doctors won't prescribe this to patients who have a triglyceride level over 200 mg/dl.

Forms of resins. The earliest bile acid sequestrants are either powders that must be suspended in large amounts of water, or tablets that must be taken with water. Cholsevelam (Welchol) is available in tablet form. Resins are best taken with meals to reduce side effects. Other drugs should be taken either 1 hour before, or 3 to 4 hours after taking a resin to minimize drug interactions.

Niacin (Nicotonic Acid)

How it works. Niacin is a B vitamin (B3). In high doses it increases the activity of lipoprotein lipase, an enzyme that breaks down lipids. This prevents them from being synthesized in the liver. It also blocks the release of triglycerides in the fat tissue. Niacin can lower LDLs by 5 to 25 percent, raise HDLs by 15 to 35 percent, and lower triglycerides by 20 to 50 percent. Additionally, it has been linked with lower total mortality in several studies. It is also inexpensive.

Who should take it? Patients who have survived a heart attack, and have normal total cholesterol levels but HDL levels below 35 mg/dL despite a therapeutic diet and exercise regimen, may benefit from niacin to raise their HDL levels. Patients who have high triglyceride levels can also benefit from niacin.

Side effects. In large doses, niacin dilates blood vessels, and it works primarily on the blood vessels in the skin. The first side effect that most people notice is flushing as blood rushes to the skin. You can minimize this effect by starting the drug at a smaller dosage and taking the pills with meals. If you are also taking a small dose of aspirin, it may help reduce the flushing. In contrast to ordinary niacin, flushing is not common with long acting preparations of niacin, which is why these are preferred by most patients.

Some people also experience stomach upset, dry skin, gout, and high blood glucose. It can also cause elevations in liver enzymes, or even hepatitis, which is why the doctor will test your liver function before you start the medication and then periodically during the first year of your prescription. Your doctor may also test your kidney function as well as your blood glucose levels before prescribing niacin.

When niacin is taken in combination with a statin it can lead to the extremely rare but very dangerous condition known as rhabdomyolysis. This condition causes skeletal muscles to break down and release toxins into the blood stream. If you are taking this combination and feel severe muscle aches and weakness, contact your doctor.

Who should not take niacins. Because it can raise liver enzymes and exacerbate ulcers, gout, and hyperglycemia, people who have liver disease, gout, ulcers, or diabetes shouldn't take niacin without discussion of these effects with your doctor. Your doctor will probably give you regular blood tests to make sure that the medication isn't causing any damage to your liver.

Dosage. You dosage for this medication will be low at first and will increase over time to help build tolerance to the side effects. Crystalline nicotonic acid, an immediate release form of the drug, can be taken in two or three smaller doses throughout the day with meals to minimize flushing. Sustained-release niacin is generally taken once daily in the evening, and has fewer side effects.

When they put me on the first cholesterol medication, I think it was a fibrate, I developed such gas that I thought I had a burst appendix. Since then, I've tried three or four of them, and they've all given me gas. Mary T.

Fibric Acid

How it works. Fibric acid (fibrates) activates an enzyme in the liver that breaks down VLDL particles causing them to be eliminated as waste or sent into the intestines as bile. The drug also blocks the release of triglycerides from the fat tissue. It can reduce triglyceride levels by 20 to 50 percent and raise HDL levels by 10 to 20 percent. It has only a slight effect on LDL levels.

Who should take it. Fibric acid is most effective for patients whose triglyceride levels are severely elevated (over 200 mg/dL) or whose

HDL levels are very low (under 35 mg/dL). Because low HDL and high triglycerides are risk factors for coronary events in people who have heart disease, normalizing these levels is an important tool in reducing risk for patients with moderate LDL levels but low HDL levels, particularly those who suffer from the metabolic syndrome. It is also often used as part of a combination therapy with statins for people who have extremely high cholesterol levels, or for people with moderately high cholesterol who respond better to smaller doses of two drugs rather than a higher dose of a statin.

However, fibric acid is not as safe or well tolerated as a statin. In one study, the Helsinki Primary Prevention Trial, fibrates resulted in slightly more "clinical events" (instances in which the patient felt that medical attention was necessary) than in the control group after five years.

Side effects. Because this drug works in the intestines, the most common side effects occur in this part of the body. These include stomach upset, nausea, diarrhea, and gallstones, and elevated liver enzymes. Less common side effects include headaches, skin rashes and itchiness, hair loss, and blood in the urine. Some patients also experience myopathy, which is a generalized muscle pain.

Your doctor should test your liver and kidney function periodically to make sure the drug is having no ill effects.

An Important Warning

If you are taking niacin or a fibrate in combination with a statin, you should be aware of an extremely rare but very serious condition, called rhabdomyolysis. This condition causes the skeletal muscles to break down and release toxins into the blood stream. The first warning signs of this condition are general weakness and severe muscle aches. If you are taking this combination of drugs and have these symptoms, contact your doctor immediately.

Who should not take fibric acid. Because this drug leaves the body through the renal system, patients with severe renal disease won't be able to tolerate it, nor will patients with liver disease.

Dosage. This drug should be taken 30 minutes before meals.

Some Questions to Ask

Once you have been diagnosed with heart disease your doctor will probably talk to you about taking medication to lower your cholesterol level. This is particularly true if your cholesterol levels are especially high, or if you already have unstable angina or are at high risk for a heart attack. Some questions you may want to ask your doctor are:

* *What are my cholesterol numbers and what do they mean?*

* *How much and how quickly do I need to lower my total cholesterol? What about my LDL cholesterol?*

* *Is my HDL level too low? What can I do to raise it?*

* *How often do I need to have my cholesterol levels checked?*

* *Which medication should I take to help lower my cholesterol levels?*

* *What are the side effects that I can expect from these medications?*

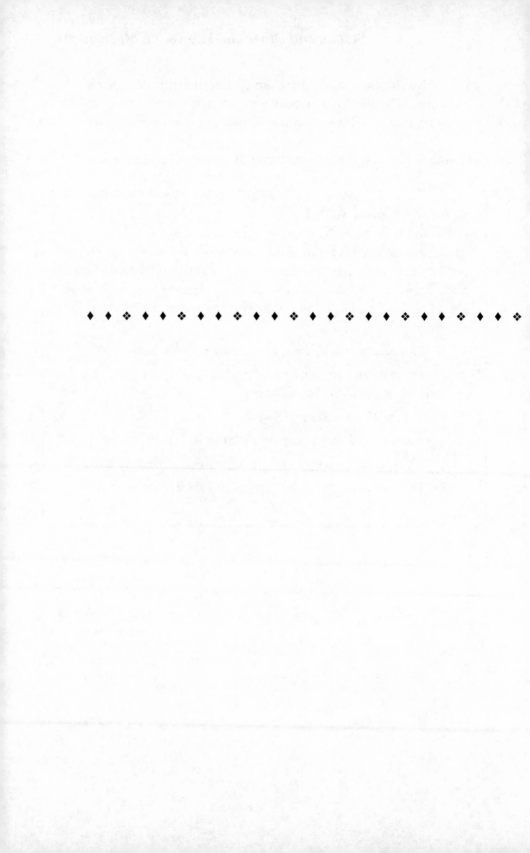

PART III

◆ ◆ ❖ ◆ ◆ ◆ ❖ ◆ ◆ ◆ ❖ ◆ ◆ ◆ ❖ ◆ ◆ ◆ ❖ ◆ ◆ ◆ ❖ ◆ ◆

What You Can Do to
Reduce Your Risk Factors

The medical therapy for heart disease described in the preceding chapters has made a major contribution to the improved survival and quality of life of cardiac patients. Beyond specific medication that targets blood clotting, heart rate, and lipid levels, there are a number of important additional treatment and lifestyle choices that can also modify your risk of future adverse events. These include participation in a formal program of cardiac rehabilitation, further exercise training, a rational approach to diet, elimination of tobacco use, control of blood pressure and diabetes, and maintenance of a stable emotional state. Some of these interventions are more dependent on your initiative than on your physician's prescription. As you will see, there is a lot you can do to help yourself.

Chapter 10

❖ ◆ ❖ ◆ ❖ ◆ ❖ ◆ ❖ ◆ ❖ ◆ ❖ ◆ ❖ ◆ ❖ ◆ ❖ ◆ ❖

Cardiac Rehabiliation
The Benefits of a Specially Designed Exercise Program

Some people who have heart disease have never exercised before, while others may have been fitness enthusiasts all their lives. No matter what your experience with exercise, you'll want to begin a safe exercise regimen as soon as you have recovered from your heart attack, angioplasty, or surgery. Exercise is one of the safest and best ways to boost your recovery and reduce angina, while improving your physical strength and quality of life. Many people recovering from heart attacks or surgery will want to join a formalized exercise and education program for heart patients, called cardiac rehabilitation.

In this chapter, you'll find out why exercise is so good for people with heart disease, and how it improves every part of your circulatory system, from the way that your arteries carry blood to the way that your muscles use oxygen. Ultimately, exercise even improves your heart's efficiency. Finally, if you can't join a formalized program, or prefer not to, you can learn about safe ways to exercise on your own.

Joining a Cardiac Rehabilitation Program

I asked the doctor before my bypass surgery, what will I be able to do after the surgery? I imagined a walker or something. And he said, "You can do

everything you can do now." I said, "Can I play tennis?" He said, "Not if you don't know how. Otherwise, sure."
Donald D.

I took a look at the cardiac program attached to the hospital I'd been in. Neat. Clean. I had never used a gym much over the years. So the sight of all the machines and the group of kind of bedraggled-looking men and women walking around in a circle with their arms over their heads turned me off. But I joined anyway. By the second visit I was really involved. The others now looked like smart people, determined to get well and stay that way. The camaraderie was great. I even got to enjoy the ten-minute stints on the treadmill and bike.
Frank F.

One of the major goals in secondary prevention of heart disease is improving your quality of life. Joining a cardiac rehabilitation program is an important step, because it will help you to overcome uncertainty and feel confident in your recovery while improving your exercise capacity and improving your health.

A supervised exercise regimen, one that is tailored for you individually as a heart patient, will increase your mobility, decrease angina, raise your HDL cholesterol levels, and improve your body's ability to use oxygen. All of these changes will speed your recovery and, importantly, decrease the likelihood that you'll have another heart attack.

Spending time with other people who are also in recovery is a good way to stave off depression and to receive encouragement from others who understand the difficulties you face.

What Is Cardiac Rehabilitation?

Typically, this is a 12-week outpatient program for people with stable angina who are recovering from a heart attack, cardiac surgery, and various interventional procedures. You will generally visit the center for an hour-long program three times a week. This will include a 30-minute exercise session that is monitored by ECG. Most cardiac rehab programs are not just exercise programs.

You will discuss healthy eating habits and stress management techniques, learn about the medications you may be taking, address how to modify your risk factors, and ask whatever questions you have on your mind.

My husband went to rehab very quickly after he got home from the hospital. He started these classes for nutrition, exercise, and medication. Nurses give similar classes for caregivers, too. I was still in shock, so I didn't absorb as much information as I wish I could have. It would have been better if they had given a refresher course later on or if they had sent some information home. You've got to pay attention to everything, because they might only tell you once.
Lynn K.

Even if you don't join a formal cardiac rehab program, your goal as a heart patient should be to do some form of aerobic exercise for 30 minutes three or more times a week.

The Exercise Session

If you have never exercised, you may be concerned by the thought of having to do so in a group or under a doctor's supervision. Actually, a cardiac rehab session is tailored specifically to your needs as a cardiac patient. This means that you progress at your own rate and within safe limits for your condition. Each session is likely to follow this sequence of activities.

1. Apply ECG electrodes. The doctor or nurse monitoring your exercise session will want to know how your heart is responding to the exercises at all times, so that he or she can reduce the workload or stop the exercise if there are any signs of difficulty.
2. Warm-up and stretching. Every exercise session should begin with stretching and light movement to warm up your muscles. The warm up helps to prevent injury and gives your doctor or nurse the chance to record your resting blood pressure and heart rate before the exercise begins.

3. Exercise for 30 minutes. This may occur with one exercise method, such as treadmill or bicycle, for the full period, or it might involve a series of shorter activities to provide variation. For example, there could be three 10-minute sessions where you can choose among machines such as treadmills, exercise bikes, stationary rowers, and stair-climbers. As you exercise, your heart rate, heart rhythm, and peak blood pressure are monitored. You will be asked to estimate your perceived exertion on a graduated scale of difficulty, such as 1 to 10, where 1 is very, very easy. Over the course of your rehabilitation, you will be able to work harder at each activity while the exercise will seem to become easier. Most patients seem to notice an improvement after three or four weeks of training.

4. Cool down and stretching. You should spend 10 minutes after your session gradually decreasing your exertion to help return your heart rate to normal. You should also stretch to help the muscles to relax.

Benefits of Cardiac Rehab

Joining a 12-week program may seem like a big commitment. You may feel that it is burdensome, or even unproductive, to walk on a treadmill, or to learn a new way of eating. Some people dislike the idea of group exercise and would rather regain their strength on their own.

The truth is that people who enroll in a formal cardiac rehabilitation program following a heart attack, bypass surgery, angioplasty, or a bout of serious angina can look ahead to the following rewards.

Less pain. Improved exercise tolerance can reduce your effort angina and make everyday activities easier to perform.

Reduced risk. Your chances of suffering a fatal cardiac event will sharply decrease as your fitness increases. In other words, your likelihood of survival improves with exercise training. Your chances of visiting the ER or spending more time in the hospital can also decrease.

Improved strength. Your capacity to perform ordinary tasks without strain or fear of another heart attack will put you on a fast track toward recovery.

Better quality of life. A formal exercise program will help fight depression and improve your confidence in your recovery.

Exercise Reduces Effort Angina

Working the heart and the skeletal muscles at regular intervals can actually improve the flow of oxygen rich blood through the arteries of the body.

What the Research Shows

This effect was demonstrated by a group of researchers who studied effort angina in 40 men under the age of 60. The treatment group engaged in daily calisthenics for one year, while the control group did not. The exercise group members continually improved their physical fitness. They were able to exercise at greater intensity, and yet each subject's heart rate at peak exercise level declined over time. Their hearts were able to support much more physical work of the body with far less effort. In addition, the exercise group members felt better. They had resumed more of their daily activities and needed fewer drugs to control their angina. The control group reported no changes in medication or activity level over the course of the study.

Skeptics may counter that the subjective feelings of exercisers may not be wholly accurate. That's probably why the subjects in both groups wore ambulatory ECG monitors for 24 hours at the end of the study to record a day's worth of electrical activity in their hearts. Researchers were then able to study and count the number of episodes of ST depression in the ECG readout. These are distinctive patterns that occur on the ECG when the heart is struggling for lack of oxygen, even if the patient feels no pain. The exercise group members experienced a 37 percent reduction in ST segment depression episodes, and the episodes they did have were much shorter in duration than they had been at the beginning of the study.

Exercise Improves Survival

For decades researchers have found that exercise reduces mortality rates among people with heart disease. Most exercise trials involve relatively small numbers of patients because these studies are labor intensive, involving exercise programs and tests, along with multiple interviews. For this reason, it has been difficult to determine from individual small studies exactly how much exercise actually improves survival rates among heart patients.

What the Research Shows

In 1989, researchers solved this problem by conducting an overview study, called a meta-analysis, which involved pooling the data from 22 different trials on exercise. By doing so, they were able to examine data on more than 4,500 patients enrolled in exercise programs or control groups. After the first year, the patients randomly selected to the exercise group had a 22 percent fewer total deaths and cardiac-related deaths as compared to the control group. The exercise group experienced a similar benefit over the control group after two and three years of follow-up.

These results were reinforced in 2001 when another group of researchers conducted another meta-analysis of more than 7,500 patients that showed an even more pronounced benefit from exercise with total deaths reduced by 28 percent and cardiac deaths reduced by 32 percent.

This more recent study also found that the relative risk for sudden death dropped by 40 percent. The risk of fatal heart attack declined by 35 percent, while the risk of suffering a nonfatal attack rose very slightly. An increase in the number of nonfatal myocardial infarction cases sounds like a problem, until you realize that it is the result of patients surviving heart attacks that otherwise would have been fatal if their cardiovascular system hadn't been strengthened by exercise. So, exercise training increases survival.

Exercise Reduces Hospitalization

Improving the efficiency of your cardiovascular system can decrease the number of times you need to go to the emergency room and the number of days you spend in the hospital in the year following a heart attack.

What the Research Shows

One study evaluated patients over age 65 who had survived a heart attack and then were randomly selected to participate in a cardiac rehab program that included voluntary, low-intensity exercise sessions or placed in a control group with no exercise or counseling. The number of visits to the emergency room in the year following the heart attack was 53 percent lower in the cardiac rehab group. Most of the ER visits made by patients in the rehab group were for serious conditions, while the control group members went to the ER more often and with less serious conditions that might have been prevented as outpatients.

Patients in the rehab group had spent an average of two days in the hospital in the first three months after their heart attack, while those in the control group spent just over five days. At 12 months, the rehab group had spent just six days in the hospital while the control group had spent nine days.

The fact that people in this study made fewer trips to the hospital is most likely due to the interaction of patients with the doctors and nurses at rehab sessions. At these sessions, patients could describe their symptoms, which can allow doctors and nurses to recognize or even anticipate potential problems. Researchers speculated that subjects in the rehab group benefited most from counseling sessions in which health care workers answered patients' questions about the physiology of heart disease, medications, and risk factor modification. By talking about their symptoms and experiences, rehab participants were better able to adjust to a new healthier lifestyle and to respond appropriately to new symptoms and sensations.

I came home from the hospital 11 days after my heart attack and triple bypass. I started rehab immediately. I remember getting on the treadmill and walking about a half a mile per hour. I was so slow. I went to rehab Monday, Wednesday, and Friday and I went to the mall to walk every other day, and I never missed a day. I was going to do whatever I had to do to get my feet back under me. I pushed myself. I didn't overdo it, but it was always a challenge to do a little bit more.

I finished the first 12 weeks and then my doctor told me I could use 6 more weeks, so he ordered that. And I'm glad he did. I continued to work out at the cardiac rehab center for almost a year, even though I wasn't in rehab.

After about a year I was walking 3.5 to 4 miles per hour on that treadmill at the highest level of incline with no problems at all. A lot of people didn't believe I could do it. Now, I still walk outside every day.
David K.

Exercise Speeds Your Recovery

One of the primary goals of your recovery must be to restore confidence in your present physical and emotional status and in your future. Exercise training is one of the best ways to keep you out of the hospital and get you back to work or to the social activities you enjoy.

I went into cardiac rehab after my bypass surgery. It was a 12-week course, but after 10 weeks the doctor agreed to let me go back to the tennis court, which is where I wanted to be. Today, I weigh more than I should, but otherwise I'm fine. In an average week I play tennis five times. I would do better if I did a treadmill for 30 minutes every day, and if I ate better.
Donald D.

What the Research Shows

In a study performed in Sweden, researchers examined the costs and benefits of cardiac rehab during the five years after heart attack or bypass surgery. Not surprisingly, they found that fewer patients in the exercise group were taking nitroglycerin. They also found that physically fit patients had fewer repeat heart attacks and fewer total cardiac events. As a result, these individuals spent less time in the hospital, took fewer trips to the ER, and spent less time visiting their primary care physician. All of this indicates that patients who stay fit rely less on the healthcare system and can spend more time and energy working or doing the things they love.

At the end of this five-year study, 51 percent of participants in the exercise group were still working, compared to only 21 percent in the control group. Researchers also asked subjects about their work capacity, meaning the number or percentage of their work-related tasks they had been able to resume. Those patients in the exercise group who did return to work had a 52-percent work capacity as opposed to a 39-percent capacity in those who returned to work from the control group.

Exercise Improves Your Mood

Exercise training in a cardiac rehab program does much more than boost your cardiovascular performance. It can also improve your mood, and instill confidence that you have control over your life and your health.

Being diagnosed with heart disease is obviously stressful. You have to become accustomed to new physical sensations, and endure feelings of dependency that occur when you become a patient. Many people experience anxiety, sleeplessness, hostility, and fatigue in the wake of cardiac surgery. Between 15 percent and 20 percent of patients experience major depression following a heart attack, placing them at increased risk for another, potentially fatal heart attack within the year. Unfortunately, this type of depression doesn't go away on its own. In fact, in about 70 percent of cases, patients who are depressed when they leave the hospital remain so a year later.

What the Research Shows

One study used detailed questionnaires to compare the effects of cardiac rehabilitation in depressed patients versus their nondepressed counterparts. They found that depressed patients enrolled in cardiac rehab improved their quality of life by 26 percent, while nondepressed patients improved by 14 percent. The depressed patients also showed improvement in depressive symptoms, meaning they felt less anxiety and anger, and they slept better. In addition, some of the patients who were initially depressed were not depressed by the end of the three months of cardiac rehab.

While a cardiac rehab program can improve the physical strength and confidence of most patients, it is especially effective for patients suffering from depression.

Exercise Reduces Other Risk Factors

Regular exercise increases the number of calories you spend as you are exercising, as well as between exercise sessions. As your muscles grow stronger and develop greater blood flow, they require more energy. This increase in energy helps you to control your weight and to burn more calories and sugar from your system. A reduction in your glucose levels will help you to control diabetes or to reduce the effects of the metabolic syndrome on your system.

Exercise also may have a positive effect on your cholesterol profile. It can decrease your LDL levels and triglycerides while increasing your HDL levels. In fact, exercise is one of the most efficient and reliable ways to increase your levels of HDL, the "good" cholesterol.

How Exercise Improves Heart Function

Exercise improves the symptoms of heart disease by changing the way your body works. Increasing your exercise capacity can:

Strengthen your heart muscle. When your heart is stronger, it pumps more efficiently, meaning that it will need to pump fewer times to do the same amount of work. But even if your heart cannot become stronger because it has been seriously damaged by disease, exercise training can improve your effort capacity.

Improve the efficiency of your muscles. Exercise training enables the working skeletal muscles of your body, such as those in your legs, to use oxygen energy more efficiently. In addition, as you exercise, your body can build new capillaries to feed the muscles and organs that are working.

Improve the overall efficiency of exercise. The amount of work that your body can do takes place with less stress on the heart.

Exercise Boosts Your Body's Use of Oxygen

The heart is a pump, and as such, it has a measurable output. The output of the heart is blood, and the rate of blood pumped into the circulation is generally measured in liters (of blood) per minute (time). Your heart's output of blood, called *cardiac output*, increases with exercise and decreases at rest.

The cardiac output of an average, healthy person is approximately five liters per minute while at rest. This average person uses about 70 heartbeats each minute to push those five liters of blood through the circulatory system. The main difference between an average person and an endurance athlete is that the athlete can move that same five liters of blood using only 50 to 55 heartbeats per minute. Is that because an athlete's heart is stronger and can beat with more force? Sometimes. Is that because an athlete's heart is larger and can fill with more blood before each contraction? Sometimes. Is it because an athlete's tissues and organs have learned how to extract more oxygen from the blood? Absolutely. When you exercise over several weeks and months, you are improving the flow of oxygen to the tissues by training them to extract oxygen more efficiently.

What Exercise Can Do for You

As a heart patient, your body is different from that of an endurance athlete or even a normal sedentary person. For example, you might need 90 beats per minute to push blood through the system or your heart muscle may not be able to pump blood efficiently because it has been damaged by a heart attack or because the arteries are so blocked that you often experience angina. This is going to affect your ability to exercise.

While you don't need to accept inappropriate or arbitrary limitations, there are some things you need to approach carefully. If you experience angina when your heart rate increases too rapidly, you can't suddenly take up jogging or tennis. Also, if you've had a heart attack that has reduced the function of your heart muscle, your cardiac output may be limited.

Even so, your tolerance for exertion can be improved through progressive exercise training during cardiac rehab.

Reduced resting heart rate. As your circulatory system becomes more efficient, your resting heart rate can slow down, meaning that your heart gets to rest for a longer part of each cardiac cycle.

Increased ability to exercise. As you improve your fitness, you will be able to exercise at a moderate intensity without having your heart rate increase as much as it did when you were not conditioned. This means that your heart can more easily tolerate extra activity that might have caused you discomfort or breathlessness prior to training.

Improved heart rate recovery. If you are exercising at your peak and then stop, your heart rate normally drops by 12 or more beats during the first minute of cooling down. In people with heart disease, the heart rate after one minute may not decrease as much, because the heart needs more time to right the oxygen imbalance caused by exertion. As the muscles become more efficient at extracting oxygen from the blood, exercise training can directly help your heart relax more quickly after effort.

Long Term Benefits of Exercise

Over time, your blood and circulatory system makes adaptations to improve the efficiency of oxygen delivery to the muscles. This enables you to exercise harder and longer. During exercise your sympathetic nervous system is pushing the heart to beat harder and faster causing your blood pressure to rise. As your working muscles become better at extracting oxygen from the blood, your sympathetic nervous system won't need to increase your heart rate and blood pressure as much or as quickly during your exercise session. Your heart will pump more efficiently, since it will need less oxygen at any given workload. If you have angina, this can be a very favorable and exciting development because your heart will be able to tolerate more and more effort without causing you pain.

What the Research Shows

One group of researchers studied the effect of 12 months of exercise training on exercise tolerance in 25 patients with an average age of 52 and a history of heart attack or angina. Predictably, the patients' strength and endurance both improved. During peak exercise, their bodies' maximum ability to use oxygen increased by 39 percent, and the amount of time they could spend exercising at maximum capacity increased by 41 percent. In addition, peak exercise stroke volume, the amount of blood pushed out of the ventricle after each contraction during exercise, increased significantly after training. For five of the ten patients who had effort angina, symptoms disappeared even when they exercised at their maximum rate. Effort angina improved greatly in three others.

More importantly, their resting heart rate decreased significantly, from an average of 64 to 56 beats per minute with training. These factors did not change in the control patients.

This study demonstrates that exercise improves the efficiency of the heart's contractions and its ability to use oxygen. The resting heart rate decreases because the heart needs fewer contractions to supply the oxygen required by the more efficient muscles during normal activity This is what reduces the occurrence and duration of angina, dizziness, breathlessness and other symptoms of heart disease.

How Your Muscles Adapt to Exercise

Even if you can't increase your heart rate or pumping capacity during exercise, it is still possible to improve the muscles' ability to utilize oxygen.

What the Research Shows

One study demonstrated this using 55 cardiac patients with an average age of 68. After three months of exercise training the participants could exercise at a 16 percent higher level of intensity and maintain that level longer (for 22 minutes instead of 19 minutes) even though their average exercise heart rate did not increase and the pumping capacity of their heart during exercise did not increase over that the training period. This is because oxygen was being extracted more efficiently from the blood by the trained muscles.

In these same patients, there was little change in the size of muscle fiber in their calf muscles, but there was a 17 percent increase in resting calf blood flow and a 31 percent increase in capillary density. This indicates that exercise causes the body to increase the number of tiny blood vessels (capillaries) to improve blood flow to the muscles, even when the body can't make any other adaptations to exercise.

In the above study, participants showed little change in the size of the muscle fiber in their calf muscles, but there was a 17 percent increase in resting calf blood flow. Even when muscles aren't growing in response to exercise, they are changing in two important ways in order to use oxygen more efficiently.

Capillary density. When you exercise regularly, your body builds more capillaries to feed the skeletal muscles, which consume the most blood. In this way, the circulatory system is able to deliver blood more quickly to where it's needed.

Myoglobin content. Exercise training can increase the myoglobin in your muscle fibers. Myoglobin is a protein that combines with oxygen within the muscle fiber and increases the diffusion of oxygen throughout the muscle fiber.

Effect on Moderate Exertion

While it's true that exercise will improve your body's ability to process energy during peak exercise, it is even more important that it can also improve the symptoms of heart disease in your routine activities of daily life.

What the Research Shows

Researchers tested the exercise capacity of 12 patients with an average age of 48 who had survived a heart attack or suffered effort angina. After three months of exercise training, the subjects took an additional stress test. The angina patients had increased their peak exercise capacity by more than 30 percent in that short time. More important, these subjects were able to exercise more efficiently at more moderate levels of activity. Tests showed that, after training, their heart rates and cardiac output response to comparable levels of moderate effort had actually decreased, meaning their hearts weren't beating as fast or as hard to achieve lower levels of exercise. These factors contributed to a sharp reduction in the symptoms of angina in these patients.

Exercise and Older Patients

As your body ages, it responds differently to exercise. Athletes in certain high-intensity sports, such as tennis and swimming, find that their physical abilities peak when they are in their 20s, while endurance athletes competing in marathons or triathlons may not peak until their mid 30s.

Understandably, many heart patients feel that they are too old to begin exercising, in part because they are beyond their physical peak. However, studies conducted at the Cardiac Health Center of New York-Presbyterian Hospital indicate that cardiac patients in their 80s and even 90s can experience an important beneficial change in physical fitness and exercise capacity during a 12-week program, regardless of their previous experience with exercise.

What the Research Shows

One study compared exercise improvements in patients of all ages during cardiac rehab. Results showed that patients aged 35 to 50 increased their capacity for exercise by 80 percent while decreasing their rating of perceived exertion by 10 percent. Patients aged 51 to 60 increased their exercise capacity by 120 percent, while patients aged 61 to 85 increased their exercise capacity by 72 percent to 73 percent and changed their perception of exertion by only about 5 percent.

Exercise and the Damaged Heart

If you have had a heart attack that has significantly damaged the left ventricle, you may have a reduced capacity for exercise. Although your heart's pumping power has been compromised by the heart attack you can still benefit from cardiac rehab. At one point, experts thought that it might be dangerous to allow patients to exercise shortly after a heart attack. In the middle of the last century, patients with heart attacks were kept in bed for over six weeks to allow the heart to rest while it recovered from the infarction damage.

In the past several decades, patients have been encouraged to get up and around earlier and earlier with good results, and it is now customary for people to leave the hospital after only days. It is also now recognized that exercise training early after a heart attack is beneficial, not harmful.

Exercise and the Heart Muscle

There are several ways in which exercise training might directly improve the compromised blood supply to the heart muscle that affects people with coronary artery disease. Although these theories are attractive and make practical sense, the evidence for some of them are not yet established. Some studies suggest that exercise training not only changes the physiology of muscles, capillaries, and oxygen delivery, but that it also helps reverse some of the underlying pathology of the disease, by improving blood flow to the coronary arteries, and

What the Research Shows

Researchers in Italy studied a group of patients after their heart attacks who had impaired functioning of the left ventricle (LV dysfunction) significant enough that the ventricle was pumping less than 40 percent of its capacity. The subjects were randomized either to an exercise training program or to a control group. After six months, the exercise group showed little negative change and even some improvement in the function of the left ventricle. The group's ejection fraction had increased from an average of 34 percent to 38 percent. The end-diastolic volume, or the amount of blood in the ventricle when it is filled, had decreased slightly from 93 ml to 92 ml, meaning that their hearts were not continuing to enlarge. The end-systolic volume, or the amount of blood left in the ventricle after the heart contracts, had also decreased slightly, from 61 ml to 57 ml, suggesting improvement in stroke volume.

The more striking results came from comparison with the control group, which had not been exposed to exercise training. In this group, the percentage of blood ejected from the ventricle decreased from 34 percent to 33 percent, and the amount of blood the ventricle could hold had increased from 94 ml to 99 ml. Also, the amount of blood left in the ventricle after each heartbeat had also increased from 62 ml to 67 ml, suggesting a further decrease in the heart's ability to pump blood. Those numbers may not seem dramatic, but they show that the heart was taking in more blood than it had before, while pumping out slightly less. These findings indicate that exercise can be beneficial in limiting abnormal functioning of the ventricle after a serious heart attack—and can therefore slow the heart's progression toward failure.

specifically by improving the function of the endothelial cells inside the arteries that help them dilate to move more blood.

It was originally thought that exercise might help new coronary arteries to grow to supply blood to areas of the heart muscle that are limited in oxygen supply. This does not seem to be supported by available evidence. Another theory holds that as you exercise over the course of months and years, the number of coronary collateral vessels might increase. These collateral vessels are the blood vessels that should be able to channel blood from areas that have adequate blood flow to sections of the heart muscle where the blood supply is limited. Evidence for this process is also limited, but even so, exercise can have important effects on the atherosclerotic arteries.

Exercise and the Arteries

The evidence is somewhat more convincing that exercise can improve the functioning of endothelial cells that line the arteries affected by atherosclerosis. Diseased coronary arteries don't dilate as they should because the endothelial cells no longer release important chemicals, such as nitric oxide, that help them to dilate. Exercise acts directly on these endothelial cells to encourage the release of nitric oxide, and to improve the cells' response to it.

The presence of nitric oxide in the body during athletic training has been observed in several ways. In some studies the amount released as people exercise on a treadmill has been tracked over the course of a training session.

Over several weeks of training, the endothelial cells throughout all of the large and small arteries in your body become more sensitized to nitric oxide, so that they are able to dilate more readily. The arteries also become less sensitive to the effects of constricting chemicals. As a result, your vessels are more likely to dilate when you are active, and less likely to constrict when they shouldn't. You may perceive this change as an increase in your capacity to exercise without feeling winded. Between exercise sessions you may also notice less angina and less shortness of breath.

> *I'm on a beta-blocker but that's never been a problem with the exercise. I work out 45 minutes a day, five days a week. I do cardio, then sit-ups and leg curls and crunches. On weekends I'm working in the garden and chopping wood. I'm 60 years old and weigh 235 pounds, I could weigh less, but I'm doing pretty well. Exercise keeps my weight under control and makes me feel good.*
> *Steven S.*

Exercise and Beta-Blockers

If you are taking a beta-blocker, your heart rate response to exercise may be blunted, and this may limit your initial exercise tolerance at the beginning of exercise training. Despite this concern, nearly all patients on beta-blockers improve during the course of cardiac rehab, regardless of the blunted heart rate response.

Exercising on Your Own

My doctor asked me to go to rehab but I found it too stressful. Maybe it's my personality. I kept looking around and saying what am I doing here with all of these old people? I'm 64, but I'm not old. I went for a couple of months and then I said to my doctor, "I'm not going back there. I've met with a nutritionist and I already know how to walk." I've been faithful about walking every night since then. My husband knows that dinner is going to be a little later because I when I get home from work I put on the sweats and head out. When we go on vacation, I always check for a treadmill. I even walked when we were in Denver, in that high altitude. I couldn't walk as far or as fast, but I walked. I'm committed. Margaret G.

Paying for Cardiac Rehabilitation

Not every health care program covers the cost of cardiac rehab. If you have Medicare, you can receive reimbursement for cardiac rehab only if you've had the following:

* *Recent myocardial infarction*
* *Recent coronary artery bypass surgery*
* *Stable angina pectoris*

Currently, Medicare will not reimburse you for the cost of cardiac rehab if you've had the following procedures.

* *Valve surgery*
* *Coronary angioplasty and stenting*
* *Heart failure*

However, the policies of individual insurance plans vary considerably. Some policies do have broader reimbursement allowances for cardiac rehab than Medicare, and you should check your allowed benefits carefully.

My doctor recommended exercise after my bypass surgery, but there wasn't any cardiac rehab center in the area. This was 12 years ago. I had a stationary bicycle in the house, so I tried that. I found it very boring, just riding a bike with nowhere to go. I moved it in front of the TV. Finally I reached for a book to read while I was pedaling, and it was my high school yearbook. There's nothing more depressing than seeing yourself at 17 while recovering from surgery. Finally, they opened a cardiac rehab center nearby. It was so much better to exercise with a group, and with a variety of exercise equipment. After my rehab was over I joined a gym, and that's worked out well, too.
Mary T.

Cardiac rehab programs provide supervised and directed exercise training that allows heart patients to progress rapidly and safely. For patients without access to a formal cardiac rehab program, regular exercise is still a critical part of the recovery process. Exercise is a lifestyle modification that provides all the benefits discussed above.

However, before you start your own exercise program, you should follow some guidelines.

I walked six miles at a pretty good clip about ten days out after this second surgery. They didn't want me to walk that far, but I wanted to see if they'd done the job.
Lou S.

First, don't exceed safe exercise limits. This is extremely important. Although there is no single way to define a safe standard for all patients, some general principles do apply. Your doctor should give you a standard exercise test, while you are taking your usual medications, to confirm that it is safe to begin aerobic exercise training. Since many patients will be taking beta-blocking drugs, this safe level of effort may occur at a heart rate that is relatively low, but your doctor can advise you how much exercise should be done to increase your heart work to about 60 to 70 percent of its capacity.

After the heart attack, after recuperation, I continued to do some running, not as serious as the marathoning I had been doing. I did three or four

half marathons. That was a good time in my life. As far as running is concerned. I enjoyed it and I miss it now that I'm older. Running is not in the cards for me right now. Instead, I do biking on the boardwalk near my home. Nine minutes at a tough pace and then I rest a bit and do it a few more times. Then about six or seven weeks ago I hit something on the boardwalk and fell. I opened my eyes to see the EMTs and an ambulance behind them. I ended up with a broken clavicle and five stitches in my head. Now I'm recuperating from that and not doing any exercise, but I'm eager to get back. I guess I'll start walking when my shoulder heals.
Ivan B.

There is a wide range of activities to choose from. You might try walking, perhaps more rapidly than usual, or you might prefer the treadmill or bicycle equipment at a gym or at home. Mall walking has become a popular activity, and it offers a chance to meet other people with similar fitness goals. Outdoor bicycle riding and swimming are both superb aerobic exercise methods, but these can be limited by weather. A stationary bicycle at home provides little excuse for skipping regular sessions.

Exercise should be performed at least three, and preferably four or five, days each week, for at least 30 minutes continuously. Warm-up and cool-down stretching is very important. Your doctor may advise that you monitor your heart rate as an indicator of adequate effort. A pulse monitor, such as the popular watch-based models that are available in drugstores, is more than adequate if you are not able to take your own pulse rate.

You are interested in sustained duration of lower level exercise, not bursts of activity, for optimal cardiovascular benefit. Do not exceed an intensity that you can maintain comfortably for a full 30 minutes; your capacity will increase as your exercise progresses. How much is too much or too little? A very simple and useful guide is that during the 30 minutes of exercise training you should train at a low enough intensity that you can talk, but not so low that you can sing.

Of course, you must be in touch with your doctor if exercise regularly produces chest pain, more than moderate shortness of breath, dizziness or faintness, or a sense of irregular or inordinately rapid heart beating. Under these conditions, it may be advisable to consider a formal supervised cardiac rehabilitation program.

> *My biggest uncertainty when I finished my rehab course was how to continue exercising afterward. I mean, should I try to increase the amount of exercise I did over time? Was I at any risk doing exercise without the medical supervision I'd been getting? I asked my doctor. He said that in the rehab program I had been able to reach a substantial level of work and that I should try to take that level with me and stick to it. There was no need to do more. I felt relieved.*
> *Frank F.*

Some Questions to Ask

If you have stable angina and are recovering from a heart attack, bypass surgery or angioplasty, you should strongly consider joining a cardiac rehab program. This will help reduce angina, reduce your risk of having a heart attack, while improving your strength and your overall quality of life. Even if you don't join a formal program, you should talk to your doctor about beginning an informal exercise program that is safe for you. Some questions you might ask are:

* *Is exercise safe for me in my current condition? If not now, when will it be safe?*

* *Can you recommend a cardiac rehab program nearby?*

* *What do you like about this particular program?*

* *What educational programs does it offer aside from exercise training?*

* *How long does this program last and what does it cost? Will my insurance cover this?*

* *If I get to the end of the 12-week session and want to continue, can I do that?*

* *If I want to exercise on my own, do I need a stress test first?*

* *What is my target heart rate during exercise? How can I best monitor my heart rate?*

* *Under what conditions should I stop an exercise session?*

Chapter 11

◆ ◆ ❖ ◆ ◆ ❖ ◆ ◆ ❖ ◆ ◆ ◆ ❖ ◆ ◆ ❖ ◆ ◆

Cholesterol

Lowering Cholesterol through Diet and Exercise

Even if you are taking one or more medications to control your cholesterol, you will need to work hard to take cholesterol out of your diet in order to reduce your risk of having a heart attack or needing additional surgery. Good dietary choices will allow you to get the maximum effect of the lipid-lowering medication you take, and ultimately, may allow you to reduce your medication.

In this chapter you'll learn how cholesterol is different from other types of fat in the foods you eat, and how different types of cholesterol either promote the build-up of arterial plaque or protect against it. You will also find out which lifestyle changes can best improve your cholesterol profile.

> *If you asked me what caused my heart attack, I would have to say chopped liver. I had a terrible diet, but I was very active. I loved to run. I'd just finished my first marathon. And I played racquetball three times a week. So, I thought I could eat anything. Now, I know you can't assume that. Ivan B.*

Before my heart attack in 2001, I was overweight, and my diet wasn't good. I used to live on red meat and starch. Now, I've eaten so much chicken, I could lay an egg. You can get used to anything if you want. I've got a margarine I like now with no cholesterol. I don't believe that fat is the thing that causes heart attacks, but you never know. So, I'm good. I'm really good about my diet now.
Jeff G.

Why Lower Bad Cholesterol?

You probably already know that high cholesterol is a major building block in arterial plaque, and therefore a primary culprit in heart disease. And, by removing excess cholesterol from your system, you may be able to slow—possibly even reverse—the progression of heart disease.

All of this is true. In fact, studies have shown a doubling benefit effect between cholesterol reduction and the reduction of coronary events. This means that each time you lower your LDL or "bad" cholesterol level by 1 percent, on average you reduce your risk of having a heart attack, or stroke, or needing bypass surgery or angioplasty by 2 percent. This ratio doesn't apply only to patients with heart disease. People who have no heart disease symptoms but have moderate cholesterol levels of can significantly lower their risk of developing new heart disease by aggressively reducing their level of bad (LDL) cholesterol. So managing cholesterol is equally important for people already diagnosed with heart disease and for the general population.

Causes of High LDL

Your body manufactures all of the cholesterol that it needs. Certain medical conditions, drugs, and dietary choices elevate your LDL to dangerous levels. For example:

* *Some individuals have a condition in which their liver makes far more cholesterol than their body requires regardless of their dietary intake.*

* *Drugs such as progestins, anabolic steroids, beta-blockers, progestational agents, and corticosteroids tend to raise LDL levels.*

* *Untreated medical conditions such as kidney and liver disease, diabetes, and thyroid conditions also raise LDL levels.*

* *You add cholesterol to your system when you eat foods rich in animal fats—meats, dairy, and eggs. Only animal products contain cholesterol. There is no cholesterol in plant products, even high-fat plant products such as peanuts.*

The bottom line is that you can have high cholesterol because your body produces an excessive amount, because you eat too much food that contains fat and cholesterol, or because your body fails to remove the cholesterol from your system as it should.

Why Raise Good Cholesterol?

High-density lipoproteins (HDL), sometimes called "good" cholesterol, behave far differently in the system than low-density lipoproteins (LDL), which are often called "bad" cholesterol. HDL actually protects your body from developing atherosclerosis, though the reason why is not totally understood. Perhaps it is because HDL helps transport other lipid particles back to the liver to be to be disposed of as waste before they can irritate arterial walls. Recent research suggests that HDL may also contain an antioxidant that can reduce the rate at which LDL particles become oxidized.

Therefore, a high level of LDL cholesterol is considered an adverse risk factor for heart disease in people who don't show symptoms, and so is a low level of HDL cholesterol. Low HDL is a risk factor that is independent of the blood's LDL levels. Regardless of how HDL and LDL function in the body, it is clear that a high ratio of HDL to LDL seems to slow the development of atherosclerosis. This is entirely consistent with the theory that LDL delivers fat to developing atherosclerotic plaques, while HDL tends to reduce it. As with a high LDL level, a low HDL level can be modified and higher levels are known to be beneficial. In fact, a recent preliminary study suggested that intravenous infusion of HDL was capable of reducing the size of plaques within several weeks. Whether this approach to treatment— analagous to using a gasoline additive to remove sludge from the line— will prove to be effective and practical in the future remains to be seen.

Methods for Raising HDL

Several lifestyle choices depress your levels of HDL. Making a few changes in your life can have a profound effect on your HDL/LDL ratio. For example:

Quit smoking. Smokers have a far lower level of HDL in their systems than nonsmokers.

Get moving. Your HDL level will also be lower if you have a sedentary lifestyle, because exercise burns up very low density lipoprotein (VLDL) particles in your system and raises your level of HDL.

Cut the carbs. If your diet is high in carbohydrates, you'll have a lowered HDL level, and this seems to be most true for people whose diets contain a lot of simple processed sugars such as bakery goods.

Of course, cutting down on carbohydrates doesn't mean cutting out carbohydrates. A study in the medical journal, the *Lancet*, several years ago, found that the effect of carbohydrates on HDL levels seems to be proportional to the "glycemic index," which is a measure of how much your blood sugar level goes up after eating a particular food. More complex carbohydrates, such as beans or whole grains, may have a lower glycemic index and therefore less of an effect on HDL reduction than occurs with simple carbohydrates, such as white bread or table sugar. Still, there are exceptions to this rule.

The Role of Triglycerides

Triglycerides are the major form in which fat is stored for release into the bloodstream as a source of energy. For this reason, your triglyceride level will vary at different times of the day, based on what and when you have eaten. When your doctor measures your triglyceride level, you will need to fast for several hours before your blood test in order to get an accurate measurement.

High triglyceride levels often coincide with high levels of LDL particles in patients with heart disease and stroke. In general, your triglyceride level is inversely related to your HDL level, but in some cases, triglycerides may be abnormally high regardless of your HDL levels. A fasting triglyceride level below 150 mg/dL is considered normal. If your level is between 150 and 199 mg/dL, it is considered borderline high. Anything above 200 is high, while a level above 500 mg/dL is alarming.

Though they are not structural fats, triglycerides are counted in your total cholesterol profile. Studies have shown that high levels of triglycerides are associated with heart disease. Some smaller studies have indicated that a high triglyceride level is a risk factor for heart disease regardless of your other cholesterol levels. Further, an interesting study published in the *New England Journal of Medicine* in 1999 indicated that reducing triglycerides with drug therapy can lower the occurrence of cardiac events. This is curious because there do not seem to be any triglycerides in arterial plaque. If they don't help create plaque, how can triglycerides encourage arterial disease? It is true that triglycerides do enter the bloodstream as part of very large density lipoprotein particles (VLDL) and then break off. One theory is that the remnants of those VLDL particles might promote the development of plaque. Other researchers suggest that high triglyceride levels might promote blood clotting.

Causes of High Triglycerides

A high level of triglycerides can be caused by obesity, large amounts of alcohol, diabetes, renal failure, physical inactivity, smoking, or eating a diet high in carbohydrates. A few prescription drugs will also elevate triglycerides including estrogen, corticosteroids (such as prednisone and cortisol), retinoids, and sometimes beta-blockers in high doses. Because a high level of triglycerides may be an independent risk factor for heart disease, you may need to change your diet or take medication to lower this level.

My cholesterol was a little high, but not in the 300s or anything. My triglycerides were high, too. So I take a cholesterol medication and I'm

more conscious about saturated fats and cholesterol—except for Saturday nights. That's my "what the hell" night.
Margaret G.

My cholesterol is good now. I'm taking a statin and my last blood test within the past eight months or so showed real improvement. It was a low number like 160. I can remember when I was struggling to get it under 200.
Donald D.

The Relationship between Fat and Cholesterol

If you have ever tried to read a food label, you probably already know that fats are not all alike. Different fats have different names because they have different chemical and structural compositions.

This may seem confusing or even trivial at first glance, but it is important to understand some of these differences because some fats tend to increase your body fat levels in ways that are particularly toxic for people with heart disease, while other fats aren't so worrisome, or may even be beneficial.

Fats are chemical substances that contain three fatty acid chains attached to a glycerol molecule; for this reason they are known as *triglycerides.* Each of the fatty acid chains is composed of a series of carbon atoms that are capable of bonding with hydrogen. These carbon bonds can be completely saturated, polyunsaturated, or monounsaturated with respect to hydrogen atoms.

* *SATURATED means that all carbon bonds are combined with hydrogen.*

* *POLYUNSATURATED means that two or more carbon bonds are not combined with hydrogen.*

* *MONOUNSATURATED means that only one carbon bond is not combined with hydrogen.*

So much for the chemistry, but the level of saturation of the fatty acid chains in the food you eat is important to your health.

Saturated Fats Raise Cholesterol

Fats found in red meats, animal fat, and dairy products (which come from animals) are naturally saturated. So are certain tropical oils, such as coconut oil or palm oil. Fats in some processed foods such as shortening can be "hydrogenated" or infused with hydrogen atoms during food manufacturing, and as a result they become saturated. Saturated fats, along with cholesterol itself, tend to raise cholesterol levels in the blood and are not good for you.

Unsaturated Fats Are Better

Unsaturated fats may be polyunsaturated or monounsaturated, depending on the number of chemical bonds they have that contain hydrogen. These fats tend to be liquid at room temperature, in contrast to most saturated fats, such as butter, which are solid. Both polyunsaturated fats and monounsaturated fats tend to lower total cholesterol and LDL cholesterol (the "bad" cholesterol), which is the type of cholesterol in the body that directly contributes to arterial plaque.

Monounsaturated fats seem to be slightly more beneficial because they also tend to raise the HDL cholesterol (the "good" cholesterol) in your body, which is the type of cholesterol that has a protective effect on patients with heart disease. These are found in olive oil, canola oil, fish oils, and in some seeds and nuts. Polyunsaturated fats, recently popular as a more "healthy" type of fat than the monounsaturated fats, do not seem to have this beneficial effect on HDL cholesterol.

Trans-Fatty Acids

There is another type of unsaturated fat that is more dangerous. These are trans-fatty acids, and they are found in small amounts in lots of foods, including red meats and dairy products. They are most common in processed foods such as margarine, partially hydrogenated vegetable oil (often used to fry fast-food items), and snack foods such as potato chips. Although these are unsaturated fats, and therefore should be relatively benign, they are not. Trans-fatty acids raise total cholesterol levels and generally tip the balance between good and bad cholesterol levels in an unfavorable way.

Dietary Changes

Even if your doctor prescribes drug therapy to lower your cholesterol, changing your diet will still be an important part of your recovery. Prior to the development of lipid-lowering drugs, changing your diet was the only way to reduce blood cholesterol levels. It is still the first step in lowering your cholesterol level because diet is the primary means for excess cholesterol to enter the body. Because dietary cholesterol enters the bloodstream quickly, an improved diet can have an immediate impact on circulating LDL levels.

> *My husband was such a meat and potatoes kind of guy, for him to cut those things out of his diet completely was really surprising. I thought he would say, "I'll just do what I want." But he just surprised the whole family and everyone else around him. And his cholesterol levels have really come down as a result. And in addition, he's lost 70 pounds. We all can't believe it.*
> *Lynn K.*

Dietary changes do work. The typical American diet contains 35 to 45 percent fat calories and between 400 and 500 mg/day of cholesterol. Switching to a diet that includes 25 percent or less of caloric fat and fewer than 200 mg/day of cholesterol can reduce your cholesterol levels by 10 to 12 percent. This doesn't necessarily mean you have to count every calorie and gram of fat. Simply by removing high-fat dairy products, red meats, and eggs (including baked goods that contain whole eggs) from your diet and replacing these foods with fish and plant-based foods such as fruits, vegetables, nuts, and grains can significantly lower your dietary cholesterol.

Even if your doctor does prescribe a lipid-lowering drug to help bring down your cholesterol level, you should still practice a heart-healthy diet. As you continue to lower your cholesterol on your

---

A Note on Food Labeling

Food labels prominently display levels of total fat, saturated fat, unsaturated fat, and cholesterol in each serving. You would think that when you add up the saturated and unsaturated fat and cholesterol, you would get a number close to the total fat. Instead, in many cases the total amount of fat on the package seems to be far more than the sum of its parts.

One reason for this is that until recently, manufacturers were not required to list trans-fatty acids on food labels. Now that requirement is changing, but it may be several years before food manufacturers must change their labels. For this reason, you may not be aware of how much trans-fatty acid is in the food you buy. A second, and somewhat surprising reason, for the discrepancy is that food manufacturers are allowed to round down levels of each fat to the nearest .5 grams per serving. This means that 0 grams of saturated fat per serving could actually mean .49 grams per serving. The same is true for unsaturated fat. So, in theory, you could get 10 percent of your daily limit of saturated fat with just four servings of food that is labeled 0 grams of saturated fat.

---

own, you may be able to reduce the amount of cholesterol-lowering drugs that you need to take.

> *My wife especially has been supportive of new, healthy diet. She loves cooking, and she likes to get all sorts of dishes and diets and meals together that are low in fat and cholesterol.*
> Ivan B.

Therapeutic Lifestyle Changes Diet

This is an all-purpose diet endorsed by the American Heart Association and the National Cholesterol Education Program that can help people achieve lower cholesterol levels. It used to be called the Step 2 Diet. The major components of the diet are as follows:

Dietary cholesterol. You should consume less than 200 mg/day of dietary cholesterol. Most food labels include a line for choles-

The Restaurant Factor

Changing your diet means making better choices about what and how much you eat. That's not easy, particularly if restaurant food makes up a significant portion of your diet. Restaurant meals provide far more food than any healthy person needs to consume in one sitting. And eating too much food is a primary way that people take in too much cholesterol. (Remember that as a heart patient, you should be taking in no more than 200 mg of cholesterol a day.) Here are some examples of the cholesterol you can find in restaurant portions:

* A single serving of beef (3 oz.) contains 80 milligrams of cholesterol.

* A restaurant portion of beef (9 oz.) contains 240 milligrams of cholesterol.

* A single serving of spaghetti and meatballs (1 cup) contains 75 milligrams of cholesterol.

* A restaurant portion of spaghetti and meatballs (4 cups) contains 300 milligrams of cholesterol.

* A single serving of ice cream ($1/2$ cup) contains 25 to 50 milligrams of cholesterol.

* A restaurant serving of ice cream (1 cup) contains 50 to 100 milligrams of cholesterol.

Don't forget about the chef's secret ingredient: butter. Restaurant meals taste so good because sauces and dishes are laced liberally with multiple tablespoons of butter.

* A single serving of butter (1 teaspoon) contains 12 milligrams of cholesterol.

* A restaurant portion of butter (2 tablespoons) contains 72 milligrams of cholesterol.

terol, so this is easy to count. One raw egg contains about 200 mg of cholesterol in the yolk. Six ounces of beef, pork, or chicken each contain about 60 to 80 mg of cholesterol. Most fish have similar or sometimes lower amounts of cholesterol, excluding shellfish (which has more cholesterol).

Dietary fat. Your total fat intake should be 25 to 35 percent of your total daily calories, but no more than 7 percent of total calories should be in the form of saturated fat. For example, if you have a diet of 2000 calories, 500 to 700 calories can come from fat, but no more than 140 calories from saturated fats found in beef, high-fat dairy products, and saturated fat oils such as coconut oil and palm oil.

Polyunsaturated fats should make up no more than 10 percent of your total calories. These include most oils such as corn oil, safflower oil, and soybean oil that are used in baking. Monounsaturated fats can comprise as much as 20 percent of total calories. You'll find monounsaturated fats in olive oil, margarine, canola oil, and sesame seed oil. Remember, though, that should you choose a level of monounsaturated fats of 20 percent, you still need to keep your total fat intake within the 25 to 35 percent limit.

Trans-fatty acids are a form of unsaturated fat found in some margarines, red meats, white breads, and cookies, among other things. Measurement and recommendations regarding limits for trans-fatty acids are evolving and not yet quantified. The best thing to remember is that oils that have been partially hydrogenated are generally high in trans-fatty acids and should be avoided.

Fiber. Increase soluble fiber to 10 to 25 grams per day. That means an increase in whole grains, fruits, and vegetables.

Carbohydrates. Between 50 and 60 percent of your total calories should come from complex carbohydrates in the form of whole grains, fruits, and vegetables.

Other Lifestyle Considerations

Omega-3 fatty acids

A few foods that contain a specific kind of monounsaturated fat actually help to lower your total cholesterol level. Foods rich in omega-3 fatty acids help to decrease triglycerides and lower total cholesterol and blood pressure. Foods high in omega-3 fatty acids include cold-water fish, such as herring, mackerel, salmon, swordfish, and tuna. Other food sources of omega-3 fatty acids are butternuts, soybeans, and walnuts. Eating 3 to 4 ounces of the fish twice a week is sufficient to gain the benefits of this type of fat.

Alcohol in Moderation

Research has demonstrated that moderate amounts of alcohol can increase HDL levels and also reduce the coronary events in people at high risk for developing heart disease. This effect seems to extend to all types of alcoholic beverages, not just red wine as previously thought. However, there is an important warning here: low doses— up to two ounces per day or the equivalent of about two glasses of wine, two beers, or two regular cocktails—alcohol can have a protective effect on the heart. But, at higher doses, the risk from liver disease or accidental death or injury becomes higher than the benefit for the general population.

Remember that if you don't drink, there's no reason to start. There are many other methods previously discussed in this chapter to raise your HDL levels.

Exercise

People who have a high-density lipoprotein cholesterol level below 35 mg/dL should add a formal program of regular exercise to their recovery regimen. It is not clear why exercise improves HDL levels, but it works in most cases and also has independent beneficial effects for the primary and secondary prevention of cardiovascular disease.

Margarines

Recently, the FDA has approved the sale of margarines that contain hydrogenated plant sterols and sterol esters such as soy bean extract. Plant sterol esters, which occur naturally in fruits, vegetables, and beans, inhibit cholesterol absorption from the small intestines into the blood. Taking 1.5 to 2.0 grams per day, or about one serving, can reduce LDL cholesterol by an additional 10 to 15 percent over that achieved by a cholesterol-reducing diet alone.

Some Questions to Ask

Changing your diet and increasing your exercise are the two primary ways you can improve your cholesterol profile, regardless of whether you are taking cholesterol medication. In fact, your efforts to reduce dietary cholesterol will enhance any medication you take for that purpose and may enable you to reduce your dosage of cholesterol medication or give it up altogether. As you begin to change your dietary choices, you may want to consider these questions, or even consult a nutritionist to help you find answers:

* *What are my cholesterol numbers: total cholesterol, LDL, HDL, triglycerides, the ratio of LDL to HDL?*

* *How seriously have I tried to reduce my cholesterol intake? Do I often read food labels?*

* *What foods in my diet are naturally high in cholesterol and how can I replace them with better choices?*

* *How much saturated fat is in my diet and how can I reduce that level?*

* *How can I improve the ratio of unsaturated fats to saturated fats in my diet?*

* *Am I ready to add exercise to my life in order to help raise my HDL level?*

Chapter 12

◆ ◆ ❖ ◆ ◆ ❖ ◆ ◆ ❖ ◆ ◆ ❖ ◆ ◆ ❖ ◆ ◆ ❖ ◆ ◆

Hypertension
Keeping Your Blood Pressure Under Control

Blood pressure is one of the trickiest risk factors to control for people with heart disease. Despite the number of treatments available, a significant number of people with heart disease cannot keep their blood pressure levels down to recommended levels. Unfortunately, high blood pressure causes constant stress to the heart and arteries, a condition that will certainly interfere with your recovery.

In this chapter, you will read about the new guidelines for controlling your blood pressure. You will also find out how much lifestyle changes can lower your blood pressure readings. Finally, you will read about the major classes of drugs available to treat hypertension, some of which have already been covered in Part II.

My blood pressure was pretty high before my heart attack, which I knew. I had no idea that I was heading in this direction, that blood pressure was that much of a factor.
Tom S.

I have high blood pressure, although recently it hasn't been too bad. I do take medication. I take lots of medication. My blood pressure is now 140

over 80, but it was once as high as you like, as high as 160 over 90, or
even 200 over 100. I watch my diet and I don't drink all that coffee
anymore. And I retired, so the stress isn't so bad.
Demetre S.

The Current Guidelines

There is a strong link between cardiovascular disease and high blood
pressure.

A recent statement by the Joint National Committee on
"Prevention, Detection, Evaluation, and Treatment of High Blood
Pressure" (the JNC 7 report of May, 2003) made several important
observations and recommendations:

1. In people over the age of 50, systolic blood pressure greater
than 140 mm Hg is a stronger risk factor for cardiovascular disease
than is diastolic blood pressure.

2. In the general population, the risk of cardiovascular disease
doubles with each 20 mm increment in systolic pressure above only
115 mm Hg. It also doubles with each 10 mm increment in diastolic
pressure above only 75 mm Hg. This supports the concept that blood
pressure, like cholesterol, should be as low as possible—but not so
low as to impair normal function. For this reason, the JNC docu-
ment suggests that people with systolic blood pressures between 120
and 139 mm Hg should be considered to be "pre-hypertensive."

3. Ninety percent of individuals who have normal blood pressure
at 55 years old would still develop hypertension as they age.
Therefore, hypertension is very much a condition of aging.

The JNC 7 guidelines emphasized that while simple, single drug
treatment of hypertension might be successful in primary prevention, patients who have established atherosclerotic disease, heart failure, diabetes, kidney failure, or who are recovering from a heart
attack, should be treated with additional drugs that have demonstrated value in secondary prevention, including the drugs discussed
earlier in this book. These recommendations are extremely important for patients with heart disease.

Dangers of Chronic Hypertension

If you were diagnosed with hypertension before you developed coronary artery disease, you were probably told that this condition could contribute to heart disease. Blood vessels forced to endure high pressure are more prone to develop blockages, which can limit the blood flow to the heart, brain, kidneys, and other vital organs. Blood vessels that have sustained high pressures can become weakened, and as the vessels dilate and bulge under long-standing pressure, they can burst or rupture. Rupture of a major artery can be fatal; in the brain, bleeding from a ruptured vessel can cause a serious type of stroke. A heart that must beat against increased resistance in the circulatory system is more likely to weaken, causing heart failure.

What Is Blood Pressure?

Even though your heart beats in a regular cycle of contraction and relaxation, your blood moves continually through the arteries, capillaries and veins of your vascular system. This is because your arteries are elastic. They expand as your heart pumps blood into them with each beat, and then they contract slightly in between heartbeats to move the blood forward.

The tension exerted on the walls of the arteries when the heart contracts is called the systolic blood pressure. The tension on arterial walls in between heartbeats is the diastolic pressure. This tension is created by the force of the blood pushing against the resistance of the vessels. There is no natural release valve for increased pressure in the arteries. If your heart ejects blood with greater force, and the resistance in the artery stays the same, your blood pressure will increase as the blood exerts more pressure on arterial walls. If the arterial walls constrict because of stress, or if they are narrowed by atherosclerosis, your blood pressure will also increase, just as the water pressure in a hose increases if you pinch it. If your blood contains more water volume because of a high sodium diet or because of a kidney problem, then you will also experience higher blood pressure.

Measuring Blood Pressure

You have probably had your blood pressure measured many times, so the routine should be familiar. A cuff is wrapped around your arm and is inflated until it cuts off the flow of blood through the artery in your upper arm, known as the brachial artery. The air pressure inside the cuff pushes a small column of mercury (Hg) up a scale. This looks a bit like a thermometer, but it actually measures the level of pressure in the cuff. Next, the pressure is released slowly and the column of mercury falls accordingly. A doctor or nurse uses a stethoscope to monitor an artery below the cuff for the first sounds of blood flow.

When the pressure inside the arteries first begins to push against the deflating cuff, there is a faint tapping sound in the stethoscope, and the mercury may waver with each heartbeat. The level of pressure at which this happens is your systolic blood pressure, the point at which your arterial pressure is at its greatest force. When the pressure inside the cuff further decreases, the sounds of the heartbeat will begin to muffle and the mercury column will stop wavering. This is your diastolic blood pressure, the minimum pressure in your arteries at that time.

I don't really have high blood pressure. I mean, I do when I first go to the doctor. The first reading is always high, and then 5 minutes later it's normal.
Dennis L.

What the Numbers Mean

Blood pressure in normal people is extremely variable, depending on your activity. It can be higher when you are active or stressed, and lower when you are at rest or calm. It can change within seconds, to become higher or lower, depending on the conditions. As a result, it is rarely exactly the same on any two recordings, regardless of whether your blood pressure is high or runs in the normal range. Except in the case of an emergency, in which exceedingly high pressures are producing symptoms, your doctor most likely will check several readings, often at different times and over different days, to get an idea of what your "real" pressure actually is.

If an initial reading indicates high blood pressure, the measurement will probably be repeated several times after you have rested for a while, to see if you are just anxious about having it taken. This common phenomenon is known as "white coat hypertension," indicating that it is a response to the anxiety some people feel in a doctor's office. The measurement may be repeated in the other arm. A major difference in the two readings can sometimes indicate the presence of an underlying blockage in the artery with markedly lower pressure.

It generally takes at least several readings of moderately elevated pressure before your doctor will diagnose high blood pressure. When your blood pressure values are extremely variable, sometimes high but often not, your doctor may arrange for you wear a portable ambulatory device that records your blood pressure periodically over a continuous period of 24 to 48 hours. The results yield representative values of your blood pressure during activity and during sleep. This can be a particularly useful tool for sorting out the problem of white coat hypertension.

In general, the numbers signify the following:

* *120 over 80 mm Hg (120/80) or below = Normal blood pressure*

If these are your readings, your doctor will be pleased, and you have no reason to read any further in this chapter.

* *120 to 139 over 80-89 mm Hg = prehypertension*

Your doctor will recommend important lifestyle changes such as improving your diet, increasing exercise, decreasing alcohol consumption, and quitting smoking.

* *140 to 159 over 90-99 mm Hg = stage 1 hypertension*

If your numbers have been this high in consecutive readings you will be diagnosed as hypertensive. Your doctor will likely prescribe at least one medication to reduce your blood pressure in addition to urging you to make all of the above lifestyle changes.

* *160 or higher over 100 or higher mm Hg = stage 2 hypertension*

If your blood pressure remains this high despite drug therapy and lifestyle changes, your doctor may need to prescribe a combination of medications to help control it.

Hypertension and Heart Disease

Not everyone develops high blood pressure. Instead, as the Framingham researchers have shown, poor diet, high sodium intake, weight gain, a sedentary lifestyle, and high stress correlated with higher than normal blood pressure. People who sustain high blood pressure for decades tended to die of conditions such as heart disease, stroke, and kidney failure. Researchers realized that high blood pressure, although it can be symptom-free, takes its toll on certain target organs over time. That's why hypertension has been called "the silent killer."

What the Research Shows

Early studies tended to focus on the diastolic blood pressure as the more important estimate of hypertension. MacMahon and his colleagues pooled the findings from nine different studies to determine the relationship between blood pressure and heart attack or stroke. The data included information on 420,000 patients who were followed for ten years. The analysis revealed a striking relationship between diastolic blood pressure and heart disease and stroke. The study found that if your diastolic blood pressure is 76 or below, then your relative risk for a heart attack or stroke is very low. By contrast, if your diastolic pressure is 98 or higher, your risk of having a heart attack triples, and your risk of having a stroke is more than quadrupled. In general, researchers have found that the higher your diastolic pressure, the higher your risk of an adverse event.

We now know that systolic blood pressure is even more strongly associated with health complications, particularly in patients over 50, than is diastolic pressure. Recent studies indicate that systolic hypertension is more closely correlated with stroke and coronary events in this age group. Other studies have shown that along with systolic pressure, the overall pulse pressure (that is, the difference between the systolic and diastolic pressures) also is predictive of future cardiovascular risk in older patients. This actually means that in the presence of a high systolic pressure, lower values of diastolic pressure add to risk, rather than decrease risk, as used to be thought.

Complications of Hypertension

High blood pressure has two specific effects on the circulatory system that make conditions right for heart disease and stroke.

Direct vascular injury. The harder your blood is pumping through your circulatory system, the more likely it is to injure the walls of your blood vessels. As you age, those arterial walls can weaken in the face of constant pressure and become susceptible to atherosclerotic blockage or even dilatation and rupture. As the large- and medium-sized arteries stiffen from atherosclerosis, the systolic pressure increases, which in turn promotes plaque formation.

Heart muscle stress. As your blood pressure increases, so does the workload of the heart. When the heart has to work harder it needs more oxygen to do that extra work. At the same time, the heart itself may be receiving less than optimal amounts of oxygen because the blood flow through coronary arteries has been narrowed by atherosclerosis. Once oxygen demand exceeds supply, the stage is set for angina or myocardial infarction.

High Risk Populations

Certain groups of people seem to have a particularly high risk of developing hypertension.

Patients with LV hypertrophy. Hypertrophy is the thickening and stiffening of the myocardial wall that occurs when the ventricle struggles to pump blood against high pressure in the arteries. An enlarged heart muscle requires more blood flow to do its work. This additional blood supply may not be available when the coronary arteries are diseased or when they are compressed by higher pressures in the thickened ventricular wall. Also, as the heart muscle thickens, it generally becomes less compliant (less able to relax) as well, which makes it harder for the chamber to fill during the resting phase between heart beats. Hypertrophy is a signal that hypertension is causing problems for the heart, which can increase your risk for myocardial infarction and heart failure. Controlling your blood pressure can help reverse this process of hypertrophy.

People aged 65 and older. Blood pressure tends to increase with age. Many people who have normal blood pressure at the age of 50 will ultimately develop hypertension in their lifetime. There is a high rate of high blood pressure, particularly systolic hypertension, in the elderly. Because older people are more likely also to have atherosclerotic disease, it is important to treat hypertension in this population.

African-Americans. There is a higher prevalence of hypertension among African-Americans. This group also tends to suffer more severe complications of the condition. The problem is compounded further by a high prevalence of diabetes and obesity in this population. In general, African-Americans seem to have a higher likelihood of having hypertension due to high blood volume than to high arterial resistance. This difference can affect which drugs are chosen for initial treatment, as well as the drugs or drug combinations that will provide optimum therapeutic benefits to African-American patients.

Pregnant women. The physiological changes that occur in pregnancy, including weight gain and increased blood volume, naturally increase systemic blood pressure. When a woman experiences a critical level of blood pressure late in pregnancy, called pre-eclampsia, she may need to have labor induced, or she may require an emergency caesarian section to deliver the baby before her health is endangered.

Women who have suffered from pre-eclampsia in one or more pregnancies are at increased risk for developing hypertension later in life. These women may also experience an increase in risk of stroke and heart disease.

Methods for Controlling Blood Pressure

Some people develop high blood pressure because they have a high blood volume. In a sense these people have more blood than will comfortably fit in their vascular system. Other people have high arterial resistance, meaning that their arteries may be constricted at rest so they can't stretch to accommodate their normal blood volume. Most people with high blood pressure have a combination of both factors, which is why they may need a combination of strategies to help reduce that pressure. If your blood pressure is high because of just one of these factors, either high arterial resistance or high blood volume, your doctor can help you identify which lifestyle changes and which medications will be most effective in reaching your blood pressure goals.

Before you were diagnosed with heart disease, your doctor may have told you that your goal blood pressure readings were 140/90 mm Hg. The JNC guidelines supports this goal for primary prevention in most people without heart disease, but recommends a lower target of 130/80, which is the same as that for patients with diabetes

---

Effect of Lifestyle Changes

When you make even minor changes in a few key areas of your life, the total change in blood pressure can be significant.

Lifestyle Change	Reduction in Systolic BP
Losing weight	5 to 20 mm Hg
Reducing sodium	2 to 8 mm Hg
Increasing exercise	4 to 9 mm Hg
Reducing alcohol	2 to 4 mm Hg

or chronic kidney disease. Now that you have coronary artery disease, your goal is to lower your blood pressure to the lower limit of less than 130/80 mm Hg. The more risk factors that you have for heart disease, the more critical it is for you to make the necessary changes to lower your blood pressure.

The first step is to identify lifestyle changes that can help to lower your blood pressure. Here are the top four:

* *Losing weight*
* *Reducing dietary sodium*
* *Reducing alcohol intake*
* *Increasing exercise*

Lose Weight

Weight is often a powerful determinant of blood pressure. As you gain weight, your heart has to work harder to pump blood to more and more tissue. This is particularly true in patients whose hypertension is due to high blood volume. Several studies have shown that weight loss is the single most effective way to reduce blood pressure. It can reduce systolic pressure independently of any dietary reduction in sodium.

Weight loss of 8 to 10 pounds can normalize blood pressure in people who have borderline hypertension or prehypertension (120 to 139 over 80 to 89 mm Hg). A weight loss of 20 pounds can sometimes result in a decrease of 5 to 20 mm Hg in systolic blood pressure, which may allow you to cut down on the amount of blood pressure medication you need to take.

Reduce Sodium

A salt-heavy diet has long been considered a culprit in producing high blood pressure. This is because sodium causes you to retain fluid. Some of that fluid increases the blood volume, which directly raises arterial pressure.

Many people have high blood pressure that's caused at least in part by high blood volume. These people are said to have "salt-sensitive" hypertension, meaning that their blood pressure increases when they eat foods high in sodium. For these people, cutting down on salt to less than 2400 mg of sodium (about 1¼ teaspoons of salt) daily can significantly reduce systolic and diastolic pressure.

Although it's true that most people consume far more salt each day than they actually need, salt reduction isn't always a risk-free dietary strategy. Remember that salt is an essential component of blood, urine, and sweat. Salt reduction must be done with care, particularly in hot climates, and especially if you are physically active. The same care must be applied to the use of diuretic drugs, which cause the body to lose salt. In both cases the idea is to reduce the level of salt in your body to lower your blood pressure, not to eliminate salt.

In people who are not markedly salt-sensitive, abnormally high blood pressure is probably caused by high resistance in the arteries. If you have little or no salt sensitivity and you dramatically reduce your sodium intake, you can actually cause your blood pressure to increase by triggering compensatory reactions in the kidneys that raise renin and angiotensin. Your doctor can help you determine whether reducing sodium is a good way to reduce your blood pressure.

Reducing the amount of sodium in your diet may seem like a daunting task, but it doesn't have to be. Most foods don't naturally contain very much of it. Manufacturers add sodium to foods as they process and package them. A diet that is strongly dependent on prepackaged foods—the ones that arrive in cans and boxes—is going to be very high in sodium, while a diet made up of unprocessed foods—the ones in the produce section—is going to be naturally low in sodium.

The DASH Diet

The National Heart Lung and Blood Institute (NHLBI) has created a diet specifically designed to reduce blood pressure. It's called the DASH diet, which stands for Dietary Approaches to Stop Hypertension. In several studies, this diet has helped patients reduce their systolic blood pressure by 8 to 14 mm Hg; and, it did so

---

Relative Sodium Content

Here are some high-sodium foods and their low-sodium alternatives.

1.5 ounces processed cheese = 600 mg
1.5 ounces natural cheese = 150 to 450 mg

½ cup canned beans = 400 mg
½ cup dried or frozen beans = 5 mg

1 can tuna = 250 to 350 mg
1 can no-salt-added tuna = 35 to 45 mg

½ cup mixed vegetables, canned = 290 mg
½ cup mixed vegetables, cooked without salt = fewer than 70 mg

---

within two weeks of starting the diet. Patients who combined DASH with a sodium intake below 1500 mg per day experienced even greater reductions in systolic blood pressure.

This diet has many of the same elements as the FDA's nutritional pyramid, with an emphasis on whole grains, fruits and vegetables, and smaller daily portions of meat and dairy products. The diet also strives to sharply reduce the number of sweets and fats taken in on a weekly basis.

A 2,000 calorie per day eating plan on the DASH diet would break down as follows:

7 to 8 servings of grains
4 to 5 servings of vegetables
4 to 5 servings of fruits
2 to 3 servings of low fat diary products
2 or fewer 3-ounce servings of meat or fish
4 to 5 servings per week of nuts or beans
2 to 3 tablespoons per day of fats and oils
5 low-fat sweets per week

What Is a Serving?

A serving size is smaller than you think. Here are some serving sizes for the DASH eating plan.

Meat serving = 3 ounces lean meat

Grains = 1 slice of bread or ½ cup rice

Vegetables = 1 cup raw or ½ cup cooked vegetables

Fruit = 1 medium fruit or ½ cup fruit juice

Beans and nuts = ⅓ cup nuts or ½ cup cooked beans

Sweets = 1 tablespoon of jam or 1 tablespoon of sugar

Increase Physical Activity

In addition to benefiting heart patients in numerous other ways, regular aerobic exercise can also decrease blood pressure. Although your blood pressure will temporarily increase during the time while you are actually exercising, resting systolic blood pressure readings may decrease by 4 to 9 mm Hg over time.

The level of exercise does not have to be punishing in order to achieve these results. Thirty minutes or more of brisk walking most days of the week will improve your blood pressure and your overall health.

Reduce Alcohol Consumption

In addition to harming your liver, alcohol in high doses can have a number of other negative effects on your body. Even though alcohol is a depressant, excessive alcohol intake can overstimulate the sympathetic nervous system, particularly in the period after the effects of alcohol have worn off. If you drink alcohol in the evenings, this can result in high blood pressure the next day. Reducing your alcohol intake to no more than two drinks per day if you are a man of average size, and no more than one drink per day if you are a woman can result in a 2 to 4 mm Hg reduction in systolic blood pressure.

The Role of Medication

The most difficult part of the recovery has been trying to keep my blood pressure regulated, even after I lost all that weight. My blood pressure was always high, even before my heart attack and bypass. The low number was consistently in the high 90s. Now it's 140 or so over 72 to 74. I take very little medicine, just an ACE inhibitor and a beta-blocker and that seems to do it.
David K.

If lifestyle changes haven't improved your blood pressure, your doctor will probably prescribe one or more medications. This may or may not increase the number of medications that you are already taking, because some of the drugs that are used for the secondary prevention of heart disease, such as beta-blockers, ACE inhibitors, and ARBs are also drugs that are used for lowering blood pressure.

Recent research has shown that determining the nature of hypertension can lead to more effective and more efficient treatment. So, your doctor may choose to profile your hypertension with a number of blood tests and trials of medications to see what works best for you.

At one extreme, high blood pressure can be caused entirely by too high a blood volume, with normal arterial resistance. This can be the result of a high level of salt retaining-hormone in the blood. The condition can be effectively treated by medication that blocks this hormone. People that suffer from this form of hypertension are salt sensitive so they can also be treated with a combination of diuretic drugs and a low sodium diet. Since African-Americans are more likely to have salt sensitive hypertension, initial treatment with a simple diuretic may be more effective than treatment with a drug that has an entirely different mechanism of action.

At the other extreme, high blood pressure can be entirely caused by high arterial resistance, with normal blood volume. This can be the result of high levels of vasoconstrictor substances in the body, such as angiotensin. One form of this type of hypertension stems from constriction or blockage of the arteries to the kidney, which prompts the body to produce excess angiotensin. When a blockage of the renal artery is the cause of hypertension, it can by treated by dilating the affected artery, using balloon angioplasty, and may not require medication. If the renal arteries are not blocked, your doctor may treat the problem with drugs that reduce abnormal resistance in the arteries. These include angiotensin blocking drugs such as the ACE inhibitors or ARBs, or beta-blockers, and other kinds of direct arterial vasodilators.

However, for most people, hypertension is not caused by either of these mechanisms in the extreme. Rather, they commonly have a combination of both mechanisms acting in varying proportion. For these patients, treatment may be determined more by what works than by science. One person may respond effectively to a diuretic alone, while another may respond effectively to a beta-blocker or to an angiotensin antagonist alone. When both increased blood volume and increased arterial resistance are factors in elevating pressure, a combination of medications may be required to treat both aspects of the problem. This is such an individualized issue that any one person's response to therapy can be difficult to predict, even with detailed hypertension profiling.

Accordingly, many doctors will start with a diuretic alone, because it is inexpensive and has relatively few side effects. Others might start with a beta-blocker, an ACE inhibitor, or an ARB. If you are recovering from myocardial infarction, you may already be taking a beta-blocker or ACE inhibitor, or both. At times, hypertensive patients can require multiple drugs to control their blood pressure. If drugs that are useful for secondary prevention of atherosclerotic disease are also effective for blood pressure control, you may not need to take any additional drugs at all.

I've always had a low heart rate in combination with hypertension. Under my doctor's advice I had a pacer put in. Now the doctor is treating my blood pressure with a thiazide diuretic and he recently added an ACE inhibitor. There seem to be no side effects.
Samuel S.

Diuretics

This was the first class of drugs developed to lower blood pressure, and it is still considered one of the safest. By increasing the formation of urine, diuretics decrease the total salt and fluid volume in the body, and therefore decrease blood pressure. Different types of diuretics work on different parts of the kidney.

A critical function of the kidney is to regulate the salt balance of the body. Each kidney contains about one million functional units, called nephrons, which filter blood and remove toxins. After removing most of the fluid and sodium from the blood to filter out toxins, the nephrons allow much of this fluid and sodium to be reabsorbed back into the blood. This is how the kidneys maintain the correct blood volume and mineral balance in your system. The fluid and minerals that were extracted are reabsorbed into the blood as they travel through a system of tubes. The purpose of a diuretic is to block some of that salt and water from being reabsorbed back into the blood where it would keep your blood pressure artificially high.

Thiazide and Thiazide-like Diuretics

These are some of the oldest and most widely prescribed hypertension medications. These drugs tend to be inexpensive and commonly available as generics. Thiazide diuretics don't have as dramatic an effect as loop diuretics (described below), which is why they may be more easily tolerated by some patients. Thiazide diuretics are often the drugs of initial choice for patients with salt-dependent, high-blood-volume types of hypertension. These drugs also work well in some patients with hypertension caused both by high volume and constriction, and they combine well with other anti-hypertensive drugs.

How they work. A Thiazide diuretic blocks some of the final reabsorption of sodium and water in the distal tubule. This increases urine output and reduces the fluid volume in the body. Thiazides also have a second beneficial effect. Over time, they can cause the arterioles to dilate, which further reduces blood pressure by reducing the vessels' resistance to blood flow.

Who should take them? These drugs are primarily used to manage congestive heart failure, reduce edema, and treat hypertension.

Side effects and precautions. Most side effects stem from electrolyte imbalances, including reduced potassium and magnesium levels. When your kidneys are trying to preserve salt volume, they may give up potassium in exchange. Potassium is a mineral used by the body's muscles, including the heart muscle in order to function properly. If the level of potassium in your cells decreases too sharply, you can develop a number of problems, including abnormal heart rhythms.

Most people who regularly take diuretics need to replace lost potassium either through eating foods such as orange juice, bananas, or figs or by taking supplements in tablet form. These drugs can also elevate levels of lipids, glucose, and uric acid.

Because of these side effects, you doctor may be cautious about prescribing thiazides if you have diabetes, gout or some forms of cardiac arrhythmia that can be worsened by low levels of potassium. Also, people with poor kidney function may not benefit from these drugs.

Loop Diuretics

This type of diuretic drug is generally much more potent and faster-acting than the thiazides, so they are not as gentle in removing salt and water from the body. Loop diuretics are very useful in treating the volume overloading and bloating associated with heart failure.

How they work. These diuretics block fluid and salt (sodium and chloride) from being reabsorbed back into the blood stream after it has been filtered out by the kidneys. The loop diuretics have powerful potential to change overall sodium balance in the body. They may also activate hormones in the kidneys, which can cause dilation of blood vessels in the kidneys and throughout the body, further lowering pressure.

Side effects and precautions. The major side effects include low blood volume and a loss of essential bodily minerals including, sodium, potassium, chloride and magnesium. Excessively low blood volume can cause fatigue, dizziness, and in extreme cases, fainting. Excessive loss of electrolytes can interfere with normal nerve and muscle function. The effects can range from muscle tremors to serious cardiac arrhythmias.

Loop diuretics are not recommended for women who are pregnant or nursing a baby. People who are sensitive to electrolyte imbalances should be careful when taking loop diuretics. These individuals may need to take potassium and chloride supplements. If you become dehydrated or have a sudden loss of blood, you should stop taking this medication.

Beta-Blockers

How they work. Beta-blockers competitively compete with catecholamines (adrenaline-like chemicals) at the beta receptors in the heart muscle and circulatory system. By doing so, they block the impulses from the sympathetic nervous system that raise heart rate and blood pressure in response to emotional and physical stressors (see Chapter 7). Some are cardioselective, meaning that they bind with the beta1 receptors in the heart. Nonselective beta-blockers bind with beta receptors throughout the body. These drugs can also reduce the activity of the renin–angiotensin system by reducing the production of renin, and by doing so they lower resistance to blood flow in the arteries and thus reduce blood pressure.

Who should take them. Because beta-blockers act directly on the circulatory system to reduce the work of the heart, they are often the first drug of choice for patients with coronary artery disease and hypertension.

Side effects and precautions. These have been discussed in detail in Chapter 7.

Alpha-Blockers

How they work. In times of stress or physical activity, the body's sympathetic nervous system releases another catecholamine called norepinephrine, a substance that constricts various arteries in the body and raises blood pressure. It does this by stimulating alpha receptors in the arteries. Alpha-blockers compete with norepinephrine for alpha receptors in the arteries and keep them from responding to norepinephrine. By doing so, alpha-blockers reduce blood pressure by dilating the arteries, which in the presence of normal cardiac output increases the blood flow to organs and tissues.

Side effects and precautions. Patients may experience overly low blood pressure (called hypotension) accompanied by dizziness and a feeling of faintness after the first dose. For this reason, many doctors prescribe very small doses at first and advise taking the drug at bedtime, when you will be able to remain lying down for several hours. Upon awakening, you should arise slowly to avoid hypotension while changing positions. Some of these drugs should not be used by women who are pregnant or considering pregnancy.

Drug interactions. Certain drugs work similarly to alpha-blockers, including beta-blockers, calcium channel blockers, and diuretics. If you are also taking these drugs, taking an alpha-blocker as well can cause an additive effect, because the alpha receptors may have already been partially blocked by another drug. Be aware that alpha-blocking drugs are used for the treatment of urinary difficulty associated with an enlarged prostate.

ACE Inhibitors and Angiotensin Receptor Blockers (ARBs)

An angiotensin converting enzyme (ACE) inhibitor is often one of the first drugs prescribed to hypertensive patients who have diabetes or heart failure, or who have a low ejection fraction following a heart attack. The angiotensin receptor blockers (ARBs) appear to be equally effective for the treatment of hypertension, and they may be as useful in patients with diabetes and hypertension.

How they work. An ACE inhibitor blocks the production of the angiotensin-converting enzyme, which acts on another substance in the blood called angiotensin. Once the angiotensin has been modified by ACE, it causes the arteries in your system to constrict, raising your blood pressure. It also signals the kidneys to retain water and sodium to further raise blood pressure. By blocking this enzyme, the ACE inhibitor maintains blood pressure and water retention at a more normal level. The angiotensin receptor blockers (ARBs) do not affect the angiotensin-converting enzyme, but rather directly block the effects of angiotensin on the arteries.

Side effects and precautions. These have been discussed in detail in Chapter 8.

Calcium Channel Blockers

How they work. A calcium channel blocker prevents the flow of calcium ions from the blood into the smooth muscle cells that are responsible for the contraction of the heart and blood vessels. These cells need calcium to contract. When the effect of calcium is blocked, the arteries relax, which lowers blood pressure. At the same time, blood flow to the heart increases.

Calcium channel blockers are very useful for reducing the occurrence of coronary artery spasm. Some of the calcium blocking drugs can also slow the heart rate, which can be beneficial in patients with angina.

Many of the calcium channel blockers come in two forms: long-acting and short-acting. The long-acting medication can generally be taken once a day, while the short-acting medication must be taken three or four times a day. The need for multiple daily doses is one of the reasons the short-acting type isn't prescribed as often anymore. People who have to remember to take a drug several times a day—along with many other medications—are much more likely to forget a dose.

Also, a couple of recent studies have indicated a possible correlation between short-acting calcium channel blockers and death from cardiac complications. There has been no such association with the long-acting channel blockers. The most likely reason for this initially surprising finding concerning the short-acting formulations is that there is a gap of time between doses when the beneficial effects of the drug wears off. This occurs three or four times a day even when the patient remembers to take every dose.

Who should take them. Some of these drugs are an alternative for people who can not tolerate beta-blockers. African-American patients who have coronary artery disease and resistant hypertension often have good results with calcium channel blockers. Calcium blockers are also prescribed to treat angina, particularly when it is caused by coronary artery spasm.

Side effects and precautions. Because some of these drugs may block the flow of calcium into the electrical tissue of the heart, they can slow the heart rate and the rate of contraction in the heart muscle. In rare instances, this can lead to a type of abnormal rhythm called heart block in patients who are already predisposed to problems because of a slow heart beat. Because some of these drugs can also decrease the pumping power of the heart, they should be used with caution in patients with heart failure. Other formulations of calcium blockers have no effect on the ability of the heart muscle to contract or the heart's electrical system. Calcium blockers are not advised for women who are pregnant or about to become pregnant.

Resistant Hypertension

I lost 150 pounds. I stopped smoking and drinking. I watch my diet religiously and I still need several medications to control my blood pressure. I'm not complaining; that's just the way it is.
Steven S.

If your high blood pressure does not seem to respond to lifestyle changes or to come under control with combined medical therapy, your doctor may refer to it as resistant hypertension. This, of course, is relative. Sometimes this is a matter of finding the right dose of the drugs you are already on. If you are already taking two different blood pressure medications in addition to a diuretic, and your blood pressure has not dropped to 140 over 90 mm Hg, your doctor may recommend that you visit a blood pressure specialist, who might try to determine the specific nature of condition in order to design more effective medical treatment.

There are many causes of resistant hypertension. These include:

* *Adrenal steroids*
* *Anorectics*
* *Anti-inflammatory medications*
* *Decongestants*
* *Doses that are too small to be effective*
* *Excessive alcohol intake*
* *Excessive sodium intake*
* *Failure to take medications*
* *Illegal drugs such as cocaine and amphetamines*
* *Ineffective drug combinations*
* *Kidney disease*
* *Licorice*
* *Obesity*
* *Oral contraceptives*
* *Some chewing tobacco*
* *Some over-the-counter dietary supplements (ma huang, ephedra, bitter orange)*

Some Questions to Ask

Now that you have been diagnosed with heart disease, getting your blood pressure under control should become a priority. Untreated high blood pressure causes stress to your heart and your arteries and can lead to progressive heart failure. There are several important ways to improve your blood pressure, including losing weight, reducing the amount of sodium in your diet, drinking less alcohol, and increasing your level of exercise. If these lifestyle changes don't work, you'll probably need to take medication. Your doctor can give you advice on which lifestyle changes and medications are right for you. At your next appointment, be sure to ask:

* *What is my target blood pressure?*
* *What are the possible causes for my hypertension?*
* *What dietary changes do you recommend to lower my blood pressure?*
* *Do I have salt-sensitive hypertension?*
* *Will an increase in exercise help me lower my blood pressure?*
* *Which medications do you recommend?*
* *Can I benefit from combination drug therapy?*
* *Do I need to see a blood pressure specialist to help treat my resistant hypertension?*

Chapter 13

◆ ◆ ❖ ◆ ◆ ❖ ◆ ◆ ❖ ◆ ◆ ❖ ◆ ◆ ❖ ◆ ◆

The Metabolic Syndrome and Diabetes
The Dangers of Insulin Resistance and High Blood Sugar

A complication for many people who are overweight is a condition called the Metabolic Syndrome, which is a significant risk factor for heart disease. In this chapter you will learn about the Metabolic Syndrome, how to find out if you have it, why it is so dangerous for heart patients, and how to treat it.

People who have diabetes are also at increased risk for developing heart disease complications. If you have diabetes and heart disease both, you'll want some advice on how to manage both conditions together, including which medications and interventions are especially important for reducing your risk for future heart attacks.

THE METABOLIC SYNDROME

I knew I was at high risk for a heart attack before I had one. I'd been a smoker for 30 years, and I was overweight. I worked as a corporate lawyer, so I was under a lot of pressure, and I drank 10 cups of coffee a day. My

doctor told me that I was at risk for heart disease. He told me to lose weight, and I said, "Great. How do I do that?" He said, "Eat less." I think he meant well, but he didn't take it as seriously as it turned out to be. He was a pretty laid-back guy. I had high blood pressure, higher than normal, but not critical. And I would get these blood tests every year and my triglycerides were always high. But my doctor said not to worry about that. He said as long as the total cholesterol number was low, that would be good enough. And I'm not being critical of my doctor. He's a smart guy and he wasn't interested in prescribing a lot of powerful medications for these minor conditions. Nobody knew about the Metabolic Syndrome ten years ago. It turns out that I have a pretty classic profile for it.
Demetre S.

The Metabolic Syndrome is a disorder related to obesity, but one that is even more dangerous. This condition is a clustering of cardiovascular risk factors that tend to occur alongside central obesity. These factors include insulin resistance with high blood sugar, high LDL cholesterol (the bad cholesterol), low HDL cholesterol (the good cholesterol), and high blood pressure. The Metabolic Syndrome is a systemic disorder that alters your body's ability to process food and turn it into energy. If you have this syndrome, you have at least three of the following conditions:

1. Abdominal obesity. Your waist circumference is greater than 102 cm (40 inches) if you're a man, and greater than 88 cm (35 inches)if you're a woman.

2. Hypertension. Your blood pressure is greater than or equal to 130/85 mm Hg.

3. Elevated triglycerides. After fasting for 8 hours, your triglyceride level is at or above 150 mg per deciliter.

4. Low HDL cholesterol. Your good cholesterol is less than 40 mg per deciliter if you are a man, and less than 50 mg per deciliter if you are a woman.

5. High blood sugar. Your blood glucose is greater than or equal to 110 mg per deciliter after an 8 -hour fast.

If you do have the Metabolic Syndrome, you aren't alone. About 47 million Americans have this disorder—roughly 22 to 24 percent of adults in the US. More than 43 percent of adults over the age of 60 suffer from it, many of whom aren't aware of their condition or the risks associated with it. People who have this condition are three times more likely to develop heart disease than those who don't. They are also five times more likely to die of heart disease.

How Metabolic Syndrome Contributes to Heart Disease

Carrying excess fat around your waist is a major catalyst for this syndrome. The high-fat, high-sugar diet that creates abdominal obesity also increases the levels of cholesterol and fatty acids that circulate in your system. The liver becomes overwhelmed by the task of storing this fat and begins sending excess sugar and fat into the blood stream. As a result, the pancreas produces more and more insulin to help clear the sugar, but eventually this mechanism fails to compensate. At this point, the muscles begin to ignore the insulin, which causes the high levels of triglycerides and blood sugar become chronic. The point at which the body begins to ignore insulin is called "insulin resistance." Insensitivity to insulin produces many problems for the body. This condition is dangerous in part because it is often the precursor to type 2 diabetes.

In its struggle to cope with sugar and fat, your metabolism can go awry in a number of ways. The heart begins to beat faster, the kidneys tend to retain sodium and fluid, your blood pressure may increase, and the HDL or "good" cholesterol level decreases.

Eventually, oxidized forms of LDL may appear in the cells lining the arteries, and when oxidized LDL is taken up by macrophages to become foam cells, you are on the road to atherosclerosis. Having any of the conditions of the Metabolic Syndrome individually increases the progression of heart disease. Having all of them together greatly compounds your risk of complications from heart disease. In fact, some doctors believe that having this syndrome is more toxic to your heart than having diabetes itself.

I've tried every diet there is. A few years ago, there was this whole low-fat movement. Dean Ornish and all those guys were saying the same thing. Hey, there's more calories in fat than in starch, so don't eat fat. Eat carbs

instead. But that doesn't work if you have The Metabolic syndrome. When you have that, your body can't metabolize all the carbs. If you're eating pasta and staying away from fats, that's very dangerous. I learned later if you have Metabolic Syndrome, it's just the opposite. You have to stay away from carbs, but the fats don't hurt you as much.
Demetre S.

TREATING THE METABOLIC SYNDROME

People with heart disease who have the Metabolic Syndrome are at greatly increased risk for another cardiac event. Your primary goal is to prevent additional cardiac complications. That means your doctor will adjust your medication with concrete guidelines and goals in mind:

* *Controlling blood pressure to less than 125/75*
* *Reducing LDL cholesterol to less than 100 mg per deciliter*
* *Reducing triglycerides to less than 150 mg per deciliter*
* *Raising HDL cholesterol to more than 45*

People with this syndrome are also at risk for development of type 2 diabetes, which can lead to a whole new set of cardiovascular complications. So the goal of medical intervention in the Metabolic Syndrome is to stop the progression to diabetes. To do this, your doctor will ask you to:

1. Remove the foods from your diet that are aggravating the syndrome.
2. Improve your insulin sensitivity by increasing your exercise.
3. Be diligent about your lipid-lowering and cardiovascular medications.

Diabetes

Uptake of glucose (sugar) by the tissues of the body is controlled by a substance called insulin, which is released by the pancreas. Type 1 diabetes, sometimes called the "juvenile" form, occurs when the body is unable to produce adequate amounts of insulin to regulate the body's metabolism of sugar. Type 2 diabetes, sometimes called the "adult" type, occurs when the cells of the body become relatively resistant to the action of insulin, which decreases the uptake of glucose.

People who have type 1 or type 2 diabetes are at increased risk for developing heart problems. The excess glucose circulating in the blood can cause vascular complications in all of the arteries of the body. It is estimated that nearly 80 percent of hospitalizations for diabetic complications are related to cardiovascular disease.

As a result, people who have both heart disease and diabetes have to work harder to control both conditions. This can be difficult because many patients rely on their primary care physician to help them control their diabetes, and then go to a cardiologist to deal with the symptoms of their heart disease. In this scenario, each doctor is treating one half of a complex and integrated problem. It is therefore important to have both doctors working together to prevent future complications with both conditions.

Controlling Other Risk Factors

If you have had diabetes for several years, you are probably used to monitoring your blood sugar levels. Now that you have heart disease, you have a host of other risk factors to consider as well, all of which are important for your health. In fact, taking the appropriate medications to control these other risk factors will be more critical for you than for people with heart disease who don't have diabetes.

Cholesterol. Several studies have shown that people with diabetes can lower their chances of suffering a first or subsequent heart attack or stroke by more than 25 percent if they take statin drugs. Regardless of your particular treatment plan, your doctor will want to test your cholesterol levels annually and adjust your medication accordingly. It's important to take the medication as prescribed in order to achieve good control of cholesterol levels.

Blood pressure. Even a slightly increased blood pressure level puts enormous strain on the circulatory system in people with diabetes.

It significantly increases the chances of suffering a heart attack or developing heart failure. If you have mild hypertension (say, 130/80 or higher) your doctor may consider treatment to reduce it to that level, as recommended by the Joint National Committee report of 2003. If your kidney function is already impaired, your doctor may want to control your blood pressure to even lower levels.

Obesity. Most people with type 2 diabetes are obese. In fact, poor diet is the one of the primary means by which insulin resistance becomes chronic. If you are overweight and have type 2 diabetes, losing weight should be a priority for you. Weight loss, particularly in the early years after diagnosis can have an enormous impact on your blood sugar levels, cholesterol levels, blood pressure and subsequent coronary risk. As the disease progresses, however, and you require more medications to control your blood sugar, weight loss may have less of an effect on insulin secretion, blood sugar levels, and coronary risk.

Medications for Diabetes

If you have not been able to control your blood sugar levels with diet and lifestyle changes, your doctor may prescribe medications to help stabilize your glucose levels. Insulin, given by injection, is the primary treatment for patients with type 1 diabetes. Insulin exists in short-acting and longer-acting preparations, which can be combined for effective treatment. The dose and form of insulin must be individually tailored by your physician.

There are a number of oral medications that can be effective in patients with type 2 diabetes. These drugs either increase insulin, decrease glucose production, or increase insulin sensitivity. One class of these drugs, known as the insulin secretagogues, stimulate the production of insulin. This class is exemplified by first-generation sulfonylureas such as chlorpropamide or second-generation agents such as glipizide. A second class of these drugs, known as the biguanides, decreases glucose production by the liver and may also increase glucose uptake by cells. Metformin is an example. A more recent class of drug, with the tongue twisting name of the thiazolidinediones, increases sensitivity to insulin. Examples are rosiglitazone and pioglitazone. There are a number of side effects, complications, and interactions for these drugs that extend beyond the scope of this book, and careful management and monitoring by your doctor is important in using them effectively.

The main point to remember is that if you have heart disease, sugar control is really important.

Some Questions to Ask

If you have diabetes in addition to heart disease, you have special incentive to control your blood sugar levels. Chronically high blood sugar helps accelerate the growth of atherosclerotic plaque, and puts you at high risk for a heart attack or bypass surgery.

Controlling your weight and your blood sugar level are issues you should discuss with your doctor. Some questions you might ask are:

* *Am I at risk for developing the Metabolic Syndrome?*

* *If I have the Metabolic Syndrome, how should it be treated?*

* *Do I have an impaired fasting glucose level, and if so, how does that affect my treatment options for heart disease?*

* *Are certain heart medications particularly beneficial for me because I have diabetes?*

Chapter 14

◆ ◆ ❖ ◆ ◆ ❖ ◆ ◆ ❖ ◆ ◆ ◆ ◆ ◆ ◆ ❖ ◆ ◆ ❖ ◆ ◆

The Importance of Getting to a Healthy Weight

*How Obesity Affects the
Course of Heart Disease*

Most people know that carrying a significant amount of extra weight isn't good for their hearts, and yet losing weight is an elusive goal for so many people with heart disease. In this chapter, you'll read about how losing even a moderate amount of weight can change the course of your heart disease and reduce the amount of medication you need to take. You'll get advice on exercise and finding a diet or nutritional advice that will work for you.

Obesity Is a Risk Factor

Since my heart attack in 1996, I've done everything my doctor tells me to do. The one thing that's not going as well as I would like is the weight loss. At one point I was down 20 to 25 pounds from my heart attack weight. But now it's just 15 pounds. It's excruciating to try and lose weight. I can eat almost nothing and not lose much. It's going to be a constant issue.
Demetre S.

I'm still struggling with my weight. If I lose weight, which I will do in time, the doctor says all my other risk factors should improve. I'll also be able to get to the net faster during tennis matches. I'm just not sure what to do after I get there.
Donald D.

If you are obese and have recently been diagnosed with heart disease, your doctor has probably urged you to lose weight. Although obesity does not directly cause heart disease, it does significantly complicate your diagnosis. It's true that researchers doing post-mortem studies on obese adults have found little correlation between total body fat and the amount of plaque in the arteries. Still, obesity, particularly an excess of fat around your middle—called central obesity—does increase your tendency to develop other risk factors such as high cholesterol, high blood pressure, and diabetes.

Although obesity alone has not yet been implicated as a direct, or independent, cause of heart disease, it is considered a risk factor because it causes, and it is related to, so many other risk factors. Several important studies, including the long-running Framingham Heart Study, have found a strong association between excess body fat and the risk of coronary artery disease—particularly among women. Other studies have postulated that women with a body mass index (BMI)—a calculation of body weight adjusted for height (see "The Body Mass Index")—of more than 26 have twice the risk of coronary heart disease as women with a BMI of less than 21. The risk for men with a BMI of more than 26 was 1.5 times that of men with a BMI of less than 21. Obviously, BMI is more closely related to obesity than is weight alone: Just imagine how a thin basketball player will easily weigh more than a fat jockey.

Measuring Central Obesity

BMI is a fairly accurate measurement of central obesity, which is why it is used by many researchers studying the interaction of excess weight and heart disease. It has about a 10 percent error rate, particularly in very muscular patients. Muscle weighs more than fat, by

---

The Body Mass Index

Body Mass Index (BMI) is a way to measure your weight as it relates to your height. As such, it provides a more accurate measure of total body fat than just your weight. The formula for calculating BMI is:

Weight (in kilograms) divided by Height (in meters) squared

BMI adjusts absolute weight for the size of your body, which is estimated by the square of height as a way of approximating body size. It is traditional to use kilograms (kg) for weight and meters (m) for height. One kilogram is about 2.2 pounds and one meter is about 39 inches. For example: If you weigh 100 k (approximately 220 pounds) and are 1.70 m tall (approximately 5 feet, 7 inches) your BMI would be 34 (which is equal to 100 kg divided by the square of 1.7 m, or 100 divided by 2.9).

Most doctors and nutritionists consider a BMI of 18 to 25 to be normal. BMI in the range of 25 to 30 is considered overweight or mildly obese. If you have a BMI between 30 and 35, you would be considered moderately obese. Anything above 35 is considered severely obese.

---

volume. These individuals may be classified as having an elevated BMI even though they aren't necessarily obese.

Some doctors prefer to simply measure the circumference of your waist to determine whether or not you have central obesity. This is a pretty straightforward measurement. If you are a man and your waist measures greater than or equal to 102 centimeters (40 inches), you are at increased risk for heart disease. If you are a woman with a waist circumference of greater than or equal to 88 cm (34.5 inches) you also have an elevated risk of heart disease. Of course, this generalization does not adjust for differences in body size.

Other Risks of Obesity

Carrying a significant amount of excess weight can affect the course of your heart disease. It can hasten the progress of conditions such as coronary artery disease, diabetes, and hypertension. It may make medical intervention necessary earlier in your life and affect how well your body responds to interventional procedures such as bypass surgery and coronary angioplasty and stenting.

Studies also show that heart patients who are obese are subject to additional risks, such as the following:

Poorer health at hospitalization. In one study of 9,633 individuals hospitalized for angioplasty, researchers divided the patients into three subgroups according to their BMI—normal, overweight, and obese. They found that the obese patients tended to be seven years younger than normal weight patients when they needed interventional revascularization. In general, obese patients also had a higher incidence of complicating factors such as hypertension, diabetes, and high cholesterol. They were also more likely to smoke.

Increased mortality. Obesity can affect your survival after myocardial infarction, particularly as you age. One study looked at 1,760 patients who had survived a heart attack. They were categorized according to BMI, either as normal weight, overweight or obese. Patients in the three groups seemed to have a similar recovery in terms of hospital complications and survival rates after one year. Then researchers factored in the age of each patient and found that 30 percent of obese patients over age 65 died in the hospital, a figure nearly twice that of normal weight patients of the same age. Another study found that obese patients of every age fare worse after five years, despite the fact that they tend to be younger than their normal weight counterparts.

Increased surgical complications. One large combined retrospective study of the medical records of 559,004 patients who had undergone first-time bypass surgery found that overweight and obese patients had more trouble surviving surgery and recovering from it. Severely obese patients had a death rate from surgery of 3.1 percent, while normal weight patients had a 2.6 percent mortality rate. In addition, the rate of surgical complications increased as BMI increased. These complications included infection of the surgical incision, increased time on a breathing machine, and kidney failure.

Recurrence of symptoms. Several studies have shown that a significant percentage of obese patients who have undergone coronary artery bypass surgery tend to have recurring angina within 12 months of surgery. Obesity along with hypertension, type 2 diabetes, or high cholesterol can accelerate the progression of your disease, which can lead to the need for another revascularization.

An Obesity Paradox

Not all studies have found that obese patients fare worse in surgery than their normal weight counterparts. In fact, a couple of important studies have found that the highest weight-related risk factor for revascularization is low body weight.

What the Research Shows

One study grouped 9,633 patients undergoing revascularization according to BMI. Although the overweight patients had worse health before surgery, it was the normal weight patients who were more likely to suffer surgical complications. These thin patients were also more likely to die within the first year after revascularization than obese patients. Extremely thin women were at particular risk for complications and death.

Another study of 3,560 patients undergoing bypass surgery found that surgical complications including fluid retention following the surgery, a lengthy hospital stay, the need for blood transfusions, stroke, and death were all much more likely to occur in the thinnest patients. The only risk factor increased by obesity, according to this study, was the likelihood of incision infections.

One possible explanation for this paradox is that a significant portion of low body weight patients undergoing revascularization are older and therefore more susceptible to surgical complications. Also, these patients may have had other debilitating illnesses, like malignancy, that contributed to frail health and weight loss. In addition, the lowered mortality rate among obese patients may reflect the bias of some cardiologists who feel that obesity makes surgery unsafe, especially among people in poor general health. These cardiologists may therefore screen these individuals out beforehand.

Weight Loss Reduces Cardiovascular Risk

Many people think of weight loss in extreme terms, reasoning that they should not bother to go through the inconvenience of dieting unless they can hope to reach their ideal weight. The truth is that even moderate changes in weight can have a profound impact on the progression of your heart disease.

Reducing your weight by 10 to 15 percent will improve your heart function, blood pressure, glucose tolerance, and cholesterol. It may also reduce your need for medication, shorten any hospital stay, and help you to sleep better. Data from the Framingham study indicate that a 10 percent reduction in body weight in men is associated with approximately 20 percent reduction in coronary disease. This is somewhat similar to the improvement in risk with lowering of LDL levels.

Of course, there's no need to stop with a 10 percent weight loss if you can do more. One study found that overweight men with hypertension who reduced their weight to normal levels experienced an 80 percent reduction in coronary heart disease mortality.

Rather than envisioning weight loss in terms of becoming thin, try to think of it as a way to reduce both your symptoms and your risk factors. Even a moderate weight loss will improve your:

Cholesterol profile. Simply substituting low-fat dairy products and low-fat meats for their high fat counterparts can have a dramatic effect on your cholesterol profile, even if your weight remains constant. However, moderate weight reduction will increase your ability to control your cholesterol levels. Weight reduction tends to lower LDL cholesterol and triglyceride levels while raising HDL levels. An increase in exercise can also raise HDL cholesterol levels, even if it doesn't lead to weight loss.

Blood pressure. Having a body mass index greater than 25 is a major cause of high blood pressure. By contrast, a 10 kilogram (22 pound) loss of weight loss can decrease your systolic blood pressure by 5 to 20 mm Hg. This change in blood pressure will happen quickly, even if your sodium intake remains the same. Weight loss can reduce the workload of your heart, and decrease the activity of your sympathetic nervous system. It can also lower the amount of angiotensin, a substance in the blood that can rapidly increase blood pressure. All of these things will work to improve your blood pressure. If you are moderately hypertensive and can sustain a significant weight loss, you may be able to reduce the amount of medication you take to control your blood pressure, or you may be able to give up medication altogether.

To do that, you may not have to reach a "normal" weight. In at least one study, hypertensive patients were able to achieve normal blood pressure with the loss of only half their excess weight. Even though this is possible, you cannot count on it, and you should never discontinue you blood pressure medication until you've discussed it with your doctor.

Glucose levels. The more overweight you are, the more likely you are to develop insulin resistance or type 2 diabetes. Men who are overweight at age 25 have a strong predisposition to developing diabetes in middle age.

As you lose weight and increase your tolerance for exercise, your muscles are able to use insulin more efficiently. As a result, the amount of sugar circulating in your blood stream will decrease, reducing your chances of developing type 2 diabetes. If you already have diabetes, increased insulin sensitivity that results from exercise and diet will reduce the amount of medication you need to control it.

Platelet function. Obesity may also increase the blood's tendency to clot by increasing fibrinogen and other chemicals in the blood that encourage clotting. Reducing your weight can restore a balance in your blood's defense system.

Finding a Diet

My husband was so careful about his diet, and he lost 70 pounds after his emergency bypass surgery. Then, about a year later, he started talking about pancakes. He wanted to eat pancakes. We went out to breakfast and he ordered pancakes. He put butter on it and some light syrup and he took one bite. That's all he wanted, just to taste it again.
Lynn K.

I spent 30 years abusing my body. Drugs, drinking, eating, smoking two packs of cigarettes a day. You don't do that and walk off scott-free. Finally, in 1993 I started having health problems. I went to the hospital and they needed a meat scale to weigh me. After that I got serious about weight loss. I started a food diary, and I still keep it. I still write down everything I eat every day. First it was 1,200 calories a day, and then I worked up to 1,500 a day. No more. I've maintained that religiously and lost 150 pounds. When I quit smoking, I knew that I would put on 10 to 15 pounds, and I was OK with that. The question was: Can I live with a little roll of fat in exchange for living? I've turned my life around.
Steven S.

This is not a diet book. There are no menu plans here because success in weight loss is not dependent on prepared meals. The truth is that people who are overweight need to do two things: Exercise more and make better dietary choices. If you have heart disease, you will want a diet that helps control the progression of atherosclerosis and helps to prevent further coronary complications. That is, your dietary goal should be to improve your cardiovascular risk, not necessarily just to lose weight in order to look and feel better. These outcomes of dieting are not the same thing. Weight loss is good for your health, but not all methods of weight loss should be expected to have the same effects on your circulatory system.

Most weight loss diets work for a while, because people start them while they are motivated, but many are very difficult to stick with. Many diets are unsatisfying, because they are based on the principle that you need to reduce calories. Also, some diets are boring, while others are very boring. This can be especially true of extreme diets that focus on cutting out all fats or all carbohydrates. Many people with heart disease are motivated enough to follow these diets, but some need a more practical alternative. Here are some of your options.

The Low Fat Diets

The Ornish diet and the Pritikin diet are the most restrictive in terms of fat, yet adherents claim that these diets have the greatest likelihood of preventing heart attacks and coronary complications in people who have heart disease. Some claim that these diets can even help reverse coronary disease, and there are studies to support these claims. The Ornish diet is vegetarian and restricts fat intake to 10 percent of calories. The Pritikin diet is almost completely vegetarian and also limits fat intake to 10 percent of calories, split up among six or more small meals per day. Note that these diets are based in well-established programs of treatment for heart disease, which include regular exercise that may be accompanied by stress reduction and other relaxation methods. These programs are widely respected in the general medical community. The caveat is this: While many patients can sustain these restrictions, many can not.

Also, if you intend to follow a diet that is very restrictive in terms of cholesterol and fat, you should be aware of a real nutritional trap that can sabotage your dieting efforts. Fat-free food still contains calories, and those calories generally come in the form of protein or carbohydrates. In fact, many low fat foods are very high in simple carbohydrates. These are foods that the body quickly converts into glucose, or energy. Eating a diet high in simple carbs, such as rice, flour, pasta, baked goods, and sugars can be dangerous for dieters in several ways.

First, energy from carbohydrates rapidly enters the blood stream, and very often leaves just as rapidly. Once your body increases insulin production and clears this sugar from the blood stream, you will feel hungry again, maybe within a couple of hours of eating. That unpleasant feeling of hunger has destroyed the motivation of many dieters.

Second, it's far easier to eat too much when you are on a diet that is high in simple carbohydrates. Foods rich in white flour or sugar don't make you feel as full as those that contain some fat, so you can easily increase your caloric intake while cutting the fat from your diet. Excess sugar in your system is stored in the same form that excess fat is stored—as fatty tissue around your mid section. That can't possibly be the goal of your diet.

Finally, if you have the Metabolic Syndrome, which is a cluster of findings in addition to insulin resistance, or if you have diabetes, you already know that carbohydrates can wreak havoc on your blood chemistry. In people who can't produce insulin in sufficient quantities, or in those whose bodies don't react appropriately to the insulin they do produce, excess glucose in the system won't be cleared efficiently and can cause many health problems, including accelerated development of atherosclerosis and kidney trouble. In otherwise healthy people, an elevated blood sugar level can increase triglycerides and contribute to insulin resistance.

The best approach to this problem is to keep an eye on your overall caloric intake. You can best do this by substituting complex carbohydrates for simple ones. Eat whole grain breads instead of those made from processed flours. Eat whole fruits instead of fruit juices, which contain a lot of sugar and very little nutrition. Choose whole foods over processed foods, even if those foods claim to be fat free.

The Low Carb Diets

At the opposite extreme from the reduced-fat approach is the Atkins diet, which emphasizes near elimination of simple carbohydrates but allows almost unlimited fat intake. This diet has been extremely controversial because it seems to snub its nose at the dietary guidelines supported by the American Heart Association, while being downright confrontational with the low-fat diet establishment. Any diet that allows high-protein/high-fat foods such as bacon and eggs while cautioning against certain fruits and vegetables is going to be controversial.

At present, a few things are apparent. The Atkins diet seems to work pretty well as a weight-loss tool, and many people swear by it (even while others swear at it!). But remember, weight loss and reduction of cardiovascular risk are two very separate things. Supporters of the low-fat approach argue, rightly, that there is just no evidence yet at hand to show that the Atkins diet is safe for patients with heart disease, effective weight loss and sugar control notwithstanding. Although this might change in the future, as a cardiac patient, you want to focus on the best evidence available.

Diets That Emphasize Moderation

For years, cardiologists have recommended the American Heart Association's guidelines for healthy eating to people with heart disease. This diet is prudent, and it is one that most people can tolerate for a long period of time. It emphasizes the moderate reduction of daily fat intake, with a much more severe restriction on saturated fats. This diet also stresses moderate carbohydrate consumption with more serious restrictions against foods particularly high in sugar. You can find more information about these guidelines in Appendix III at the end of this book. The Therapeutic Lifestyle Changes diet is also detailed in Chapter 11.

The "South Beach" diet has achieved popularity as a weight-loss program, and has been referred to as an Atkins-type diet. However, at its core it has much more in common with the AHA guidelines. It is a non-vegetarian, heart-healthy diet that involves moderate fat restriction. Like the Atkins diet, the South Beach diet begins with extreme carbohydrate restriction for an initial period. Unlike Atkins, this diet allows the re-introduction of moderate amounts of complex carbohydrates. In its maintenance phase, the South Beach diet may be more restrictive of carbohydrates than the AHA diet guidelines, but like AHA, it advises moderation in both fat and carbohydrates.

The Role of Exercise

Exercise is a wonderful, all-purpose tool for improving metabolism. It has a positive effect on your blood pressure, blood sugar, and cholesterol levels. It improves your circulation, gives you more energy, lowers your resting heart rate, and helps you sleep at night. When combined with a sensible diet, physical activity can also help you to lose weight. The exercise you choose doesn't need to be grueling to give you all of these benefits. Just 30 to 45 minutes of vigorous walking every day can help you control your weight and improve your health. Weight loss associated with activity does not occur simply from burning more calories during the time you exercise. Exercise is also known to increase basal metabolism, which means that your body burns more calories even when you are between exercise sessions. In effect, your metabolism is activated all day and night long by regular periods of exercise. This leads to a very desirable and powerful effect, which is essentially "free" weight reduction for most of the day.

Medications to Treat Obesity

If you are severely obese and have been unable to reduce your weight with diet and exercise alone, your doctor may prescribe weight loss medication. There are several types of medications that can assist in weight loss. Some act by blocking the absorption of fat from your intestines. Others affect brain chemicals that control appetite. Interesting recent research has identified a protein, called leptin, that seems to play a role in the regulation of appetite and energy metabolism. Inadequate levels of leptin, and relative resistance to leptin, may explain rare causes of obesity in humans. These findings may lead to new approaches to the treatment of obesity in the future. At present, before considering weight-loss medication, you should talk to your doctor about the benefits and side effects of the drugs that are available.

Some years ago, it was not uncommon for some doctors to prescribe stimulant drugs, such as amphetamines, for weight loss. This medication mimics the chemicals released by the sympathetic nervous system in the body. By doing so, these drugs increase in heart rate, blood pressure, and stress in the heart, all of which can be extremely dangerous in patients with heart disease. Don't use them.

Thyroid hormone increases your metabolism and can lead to

weight loss. Indeed, one of the symptoms of abnormally high thyroid production by the body is unexplained loss of body weight, while deficiency of thyroid hormone is often associated with marked weight gain. In the past, some doctors would prescribe this hormone as an aid to weight loss in people whose thyroid function was not underactive. This practice is now considered to be hazardous in patients with heart disease, since thyroid hormone can speed the heart rate, provoke arrhythmias, and increase blood pressure. If you have heart disease and are already taking thyroid hormone replacement for an underactive thyroid gland, be sure that your replacement levels match your needs. You'll need regular blood tests to make sure you are taking the right amount.

SURGERY FOR OBESITY

Some extremely obese people who have not been able to control their weight with diet, exercise, or medication may be candidates for surgical procedures that cut out part of the digestive tract to reduce food absorption by the body. Obviously, this is not a first-line approach to weight reduction. Individuals considering these procedures must discuss the details with their doctors. All surgery has risks and side effects. Reducing food absorption can lead to vitamin and mineral deficiencies. But, for the right patients, these procedures may be effective and even life-saving.

Some Questions to Ask

Carrying an excess of body fat holds special risks for people with heart disease. Primarily, it makes many other risk factors, including blood pressure, glucose levels and cholesterol levels harder to control, which means you may need more medication to treat these conditions. By contrast, losing even a moderate amount of weight can make a huge difference in your overall health and can help slow the progress of atherosclerosis. Here are some issues to discuss with your doctor.

* *What is my BMI?*

* *Which dietary changes would help me to control my weight?*

* *What exercise regimen might help me to reduce my weight?*

* *Do I need to see a nutritionist to find out why past diets have failed?*

* *Are there any medications that might help me to lose weight?*

Chapter 15

♦ ❖ ♦ ♦ ❖ ♦ ♦ ❖ ♦ ♦ ❖ ♦ ♦ ❖ ♦ ♦ ❖ ♦ ♦

Choosing Life over Smoking:
How Smoking Hurts Your Heart

The last thing most smokers want to hear is that they need to quit in order to improve their health. Unfortunately, if you have recently been diagnosed with heart disease, this is likely to be the first piece of advice your doctor gives you, particularly if you've had a heart attack or bypass surgery. Numerous studies have shown that giving up cigarettes improves your risk profile dramatically. In fact, if you can quit and stick to it for just two years, you may be able to reduce your risk of having another coronary event to that of someone who has never smoked.

In this chapter, you'll gain incentive to quit. You'll find out how your pattern of tobacco use can help you find a method for quitting that works best for you. You'll also get some concrete strategies for getting through those first few days and weeks. Finally, you'll read about medications such as nicotine replacement therapy that may help you quit.

It's easy to stop smoking. The hard part is staying stopped. I've quit for a week, a month, an hour, but never really stopped. One time I was in Spain. I'd quit smoking a couple of months before and I was on a bus that was waiting at a stoplight. I looked out the window and saw some-

one on the street light up a cigarette and take that first puff. I couldn't wait to get off that bus and smoke a cigarette.
Steven S.

I've watched guys smoke through their tracheotomy tubes. It seems like a fast way to go if the tank catches.
Lou S.

Why Quitting Is So Hard

According to statistics gathered by the American Cancer Society, nearly 70 percent of smokers say they want to quit. A significant number of those have attempted to quit and failed to do so; many have tried several times. This rate of failure is not surprising when you consider that nicotine is a powerful drug and that a cigarette is a product designed specifically to encourage physiological addiction because it delivers a fairly high dose of nicotine directly into the blood stream. If you smoke, you probably also experience a psychological addiction—the feeling that you need a cigarette in times of stress, fear, anger and depression. On top of that, smoking may have become a ritual associated with certain times of the day or certain friends. All of these factors combine to anchor the smoking habit in your life, making it more difficult to quit.

Why Quitting Is So Important

Despite the difficulties you face, quitting smoking is the most important thing you can do to improve your cardiovascular system and your chances of survival if you have coronary artery disease. If you stop smoking, you can decrease your relative risk of a heart attack by 30 percent to 60 percent. This one action trumps all other interventions by a wide margin.

On the other hand, if you continue to smoke, the cigarettes will raise your cholesterol and blood pressure, and accelerate the development of arterial plaque. Not only will smoking hinder your efforts to exercise, but it will also interfere with the effectiveness of your beta-blocker medication.

If you are scheduled for a bypass or revascularization, or have survived a heart attack, now is the time to quit. If you have survived an episode of unstable angina, giving up cigarettes should be your top priority. Unstable angina is often a warning of an impending heart attack. In this situation, the supply of oxygen to your heart is particularly sensitive to the adverse effects of cigarette smoke. Continuing to smoke can cause arterial plaque to rupture, and it can increase your blood's tendency to clot. It can also promote arrhythmias that will contribute to a heart attack or cardiac arrest. By quitting smoking now, you will reduce your short-term and long-term risks for suffering a potentially fatal heart attack.

How Smoking Hurts Your Heart

I was in my doctor's office. He was giving me prescriptions for my beta-blocker, my water pill, my blood pressure medication, my cholesterol medication. All these pills. He handed them over and said, "You quit smoking, right?" I said, "No. Not really." The doctor took all my prescriptions away from me. He said, "You'll be dead of a stroke in six months, so I'm not going to waste your time with these." He threw them all away. I saw my wife's face as clearly as if she were in the room and I thought, I don't want to die and leave her. So I took my pack of cigarettes out and threw them away in front of the doctor. I told him I'd never smoke again. He took them out of the garbage can and handed them back. He said he didn't believe me. Then he said, "If you're serious, I'll give you a prescription for the gum." I filled that prescription. I had a pack of gum in my car, one in my home and one in my office, but I never chewed a piece. And I never had another cigarette again. That was four years ago.
Steven S.

Nicotine is a psychoactive drug, which means that it acts directly on the brain. Because smoking injects nicotine into the blood stream directly from the lungs, it takes effect rapidly. Smoking causes the central nervous system to release the chemicals, norepinephrine and dopamine, which are collectively known as neurotransmitters. The norepinephrine makes you feel more alert while the dopamine makes you feel more relaxed. If you are a real smoker, you can unconsciously regulate the effect of nicotine to produce either stimulation or relaxation.

Of course, these are not the only physical effects that nicotine and cigarette smoke have on the body. The drug's effects on your heart, lungs, blood, blood vessels, and cholesterol are the ones that damage your cardiovascular system. These effects are dose dependent, which means that someone who smokes more than 25 cigarettes per day is more than five times as likely as a nonsmoker to die from heart disease. But even rare cigarette use is dangerous. The same goes for cigars and pipes, and also for chewing tobacco. Even without inhaling, nicotine is rapidly absorbed from the tissues of the mouth. Of course, there's also the tar and cancer-causing chemicals, but let's focus on the nicotine.

Nicotine's Effects on Your Body

Increased heart rate. Nicotine can make your heart pound. Even though this effect lasts only a few minutes, an elevated heart rate is especially dangerous to you because it increases your heart's need for oxygen while decreasing its supply. During every heartbeat, the arteries that feed oxygen-rich blood to the heart muscle are compressed by the heart's contraction. In effect, your heart muscle uses the pause in between beats to process its own oxygen. For someone with heart disease, each pause between heartbeats is critical for your heart's continued health. Smoking a cigarette and increasing that heart rate will stress your heart and may cause angina or ischemia.

If you suffered a serious heart attack in which much of the cardiac muscle was damaged, or if you have the first signs of heart failure, meaning your ventricles don't work as efficiently as they should, this increased heart rate is especially dangerous. It can aggravate potentially fatal arrhythmias. What's worse, you are directly counteracting the effects of your beta-blocker, which is supposed to be keeping your heart rate under control.

Increased blood pressure. Nicotine is a vasoconstrictor, meaning that it increases the tension of arterial blood vessels, particularly the smaller ones that feed your body's tissues and organs, including the heart. You may notice nicotine's effects primarily in your extremities, such as cold hands and feet. Some people are more sensitive to this effect than others. Decreasing blood flow in the small vessels increases blood pressure, which works against the effects of your blood pressure medication and increases your heart's workload. The resulting high blood pressure can also accelerate atherosclerosis because the fast-moving, highly pressurized blood flow is more likely to damage the arteries and lay the groundwork for plaque to develop.

Decreased oxygen supply. Cigarettes deliver nicotine into the blood stream in the smoke that uses the same path traveled by the oxygen you breathe. Oxygen molecules bind to hemoglobin in the red blood cells, and that's how oxygen is carried through your system. When you smoke a cigarette, carbon monoxide in the smoke binds to some of the hemoglobin and gets carried through your system instead of oxygen. (Yes, carbon monoxide, the same stuff that is in air pollution and exhaust fumes.) Immediately, you are taking in less oxygen than your body is used to. To compensate, your heart pumps harder and faster to deliver more oxygen.

In addition, nicotine constricts your bronchioles, the tiny tubes that bring air into the tissues of the lungs where oxygen can be extracted. Narrowing these airways immediately reduces the amount of oxygen coming into your system. At the same time, the cigarette smoke irritates the tissues inside your lungs and causes fluids and mucus to collect. The smoke also immobilizes and can damage the hair-like cilia that line the tissues inside the lungs. Normally the cilia are moving continuously to push mucus and foreign particles up and out of the lungs. Without the movement of cilia, the lungs can't clean themselves, and the debris and fluid that collects inside them further interferes with oxygen intake.

If you are still smoking, keep reading. These factors—increased heart rate, increased blood pressure, and decreased oxygen availability—explain why smokers tend to be on average ten years younger than nonsmokers when they have their first heart attack. It also explains why smoking has such a pronounced effect on people suffering from unstable angina or acute myocardial infarction. In both of these conditions, oxygen supply to the heart is critical, and cigarette smoking reduces that supply.

Reduced "good" cholesterol. Smoking also decreases the amount of HDL or good cholesterol in your system. Having a low HDL cholesterol level is itself a risk factor for heart disease, particularly if your LDL or bad cholesterol level is high.

Increased blood clotting. Nicotine and other toxins in cigarette smoke enter the blood stream and irritate the endothelial cells, which promotes atherosclerosis. This is why smoking after a bypass can quickly negate the value of the surgery; it can hasten the blockage of the bypass artery or vein.

Nicotine can also partially counteract the effects of aspirin or anticoagulants you may be taking to prevent clotting. This is because it increases the amount of fibrinogen in your system, which is one of the substances that creates blood clots.

Long-Term Risks of Smoking

These negative effects on the cardiovascular system have a long-term effect on survival. Researchers interviewed a group of 498 patients under the age of 60 who had survived either a first episode of unstable angina or a heart attack two years earlier. The researchers followed this group for an additional 13 years and found that those who continued to smoke had a significantly higher mortality rate (above 82 percent) than those patients who stopped smoking (37 percent). The mortality rate was highest among smokers with unstable angina. Their risk of dying was five times as great as patients who quit smoking.

Quitting Reduces Your Risk

While giving up cigarettes has long-term benefits such as decreasing your chances of having another heart attack, needing a revascularization procedure, and dying from heart disease, it also brings more immediate improvements in your health. In fact, several studies have shown that no matter how much you smoke or for how long you have smoked, you can sharply decrease the negative cardiovascular effects of smoking within a couple of years after you quit. Within days of quitting smoking you can also reduce the likelihood of suffering fatal arrhythmias, which are markedly increased by tobacco.

What the Research Shows

One study followed a group of 2,619 people after their first heart attack, dividing the patients into four groups: those who were active smokers, those who had quit smoking at the time of their heart attack, those who had quit before their heart attack, and those who had never smoked. Not surprisingly, they found that people who continued to smoke after their heart attack were 50 percent more likely to suffer another coronary event than nonsmokers. On the other hand, people who quit and stayed quit for three years were no more likely to suffer another heart attack than people who had *never* smoked.

Researchers found similar results in another study of 1,873 men under the age of 55. The relative risk for a heart attack for those who were current smokers was nearly three times as great as nonsmokers. The risk for those who had quit less than two years previously was twice as great as nonsmokers, while the relative risk for those who had quit smoking more than two years before was exactly the same as that of nonsmokers of the same age. This was true regardless of the number of packs per day that they smoked and the number of years they had been smoking. This was also true regardless of the number of other risk factors present.

How Quickly Will Your Health Improve?

According to the American Cancer Society's Fresh Start Program, your health begins to improve within minutes of your last cigarette.

Within 20 minutes. Your pulse slows to a more normal rate and your blood pressure goes down. The circulation to your hands and feet improves, returning them to a normal temperature.

After 8 hours. The abnormal level of carbon monoxide in your blood is reduced, which allows the oxygen level in your blood to increase.

After 24 hours. Your chances of dying from a heart attack begin to decrease.

Within 48 hours. The nerve endings in your nose and mouth that regulate taste and smell become more sensitive. As a result, your ability to smell and taste food improves.

After 72 hours. Your bronchial tubes relax, making it easier to breathe.

After 2 weeks. Walking becomes easier for you as your circulation improves. By now your lung function may have improved by as much as 30 percent.

From 1 to 9 months. Cilia begin to function more normally in the lungs, increasing your body's ability to handle mucus, clean the lungs, and prevent infection. As a result, coughing, sinus congestion, fatigue, and shortness of breath all decrease, while your body's overall energy level increases.

After 5 years. Your chances of dying from lung cancer are cut in half.

At 10 years. Your risk of lung cancer is almost as low as for people who never smoked, and so is your relative risk of heart disease. Your risk of other cancers, including those of the mouth, larynx, kidney, bladder, and pancreas have all decreased.

Quitting Makes Other Interventions Much More Effective

At this point, you may be bargaining with yourself, arguing that maybe you can keep smoking as long as you do everything else your doctor prescribes. You may think that you can work hard to control your diabetes, your blood pressure, your cholesterol, or that you can begin exercising and taking the beta-blocker, the ACE inhibitor, and the daily aspirin. You may think that if you do all of these things, you can allow yourself to smoke and that it will be okay.

That is a bad bargain.

The truth is that removing nicotine and the other elements in cigarette smoke from your system will make all of the other risk factors easier to control, while increasing the effectiveness of your medications. Your blood pressure will go down; your insulin sensitivity will improve (that is, your insulin resistance will decrease); your lungs and muscles will be better able to handle exercise; your cholesterol numbers will improve; and the rate at which your arteries narrow will slow down.

Women and Smoking

According to statistics gathered by the American Heart Association, about 20 percent of American women currently smoke, compared to 25 percent of men. Some women still feel that low tar and nicotine brands of cigarettes are somehow less toxic than regular cigarettes. Unfortunately, this is probably not true.

Regardless of the type or brand of cigarette you smoke, the risk of myocardial infarction is the same. More important, you should know that as a woman who smokes your risk of a heart attack or other coronary event may be worse than that of a man who smokes.

One study that interviewed women about their smoking habits after they had survived their first heart attack found that women who smoke are three times more likely to suffer a first myocardial infarction than someone their age who has never smoked. If you are a woman who smokes more than 25 cigarettes a day, you are nearly five times more likely to suffer a first heart attack than a nonsmoker. (A man who smokes more than 25 cigarettes a day, and has smoked for more than 20 years is a little more than four times more likely to suffer a first heart attack than a nonsmoker his age.) You are more than seven times more likely to have that first heart attack if you smoke more than 35 cigarettes a day.

The good news, again, is that your risk declines very quickly after you quit. After two years of abstinence, your risk of suffering a coronary event shrinks to near normal levels for nonsmokers, regardless of how many years you were a smoker or how many cigarettes per day you smoked.

Smoking after Myocardial Infarction

Among people who have survived a heart attack, there are some clear differences between smokers and nonsmokers. Smokers don't have as much atherosclerosis when they suffer their first heart attack. They also don't have as many risk factors that will put them in the path of coronary events, and they tend to be younger. In short, their coronary artery disease isn't as severe as the average nonsmoker who suffers a first heart attack. Yet they still have had a heart attack. Why? Primarily because smokers have higher blood pressure, more blood clots, and an already reduced oxygen flow to the heart muscle. The cause of the heart attack in these patients is often a blood clot in an artery that may be only moderately narrowed by plaque.

If you are a smoker who has survived a first heart attack, this should be important news. By changing one factor in your life, you can dramatically improve your overall health and drastically reduce the chances that you will have to go through this again. Smokers

---

What the Research Shows

One study followed a group of 456 patients who had survived heart attack with the help of thrombolytic (clot busting) drugs. The patients were interviewed to determine their smoking status and other risk factors. After 12 months, the researchers found that smoking was the risk factor most predictive of another coronary event. Twenty percent of patients who continued to smoke had another heart attack compared with 5.1 percent of those who stopped. A similar study found that long-term survival improves among nonsmokers. Four years after their heart attack, those who quit smoking had a mortality rate of 17 percent while the mortality rate among those who continued to smoke was 31 percent.

who quit after their first heart attack have a similar risk for suffering another coronary event as nonsmokers who have never had a heart attack.

By contrast, if you continue to smoke, your chances of suffering another heart attack are almost three times higher than your non-smoking counterpart, regardless of your other risk factors. Many patients stop smoking when they are hospitalized for coronary disease. In fact, there is nothing like a stay in the coronary care unit to discourage smoking, at least temporarily.

People who stop smoking after their heart attack have an easier time in recovery. They report fewer symptoms of chest pain, nausea, headache, and dizziness compared to those who continue to smoke in the first year following hospitalization.

> *I was in the emergency room before my bypass and went into the bathroom and I snuck a cigarette with my wife yelling at me from outside the door. I should probably have known better. My dad smoked, and after he had his heart transplant, the years of smoking got to him. That was the thing that made him so miserable. He suddenly had a healthy heart, but his lungs were still full of tar.*
> *Lou S.*

> *My husband had always been healthy. The worst thing he did was smoking. He did sneak a cigarette in the emergency room bathroom. I was so angry with him, even though I did understand because I had smoked, too. He did quit smoking after his first bypass, and it has been 12 years since.*
> *Denise S., Lou's wife*

Dangers of Smoking after Bypass Surgery

Smoking is especially dangerous to patients who have undergone coronary artery bypass grafts (CABG). While atherosclerosis in your coronary arteries took decades to develop, this same disease can build in the vein grafts used to circumvent blockages in just a few years. Smoking accelerates the growth of arterial plaque in the new bypass vessel and continues the process in the remaining native arteries, which means that it increases the likelihood of another bypass surgery or angioplasty.

In several studies, researchers have found that people who continue to smoke after bypass surgery double their relative risk of death and increase their risk for a nonfatal heart attack and angina. In fact, the patients' smoking status was one of the strongest predictors of future coronary events.

For many people emergency bypass surgery is the impetus they need for giving up cigarettes. Spending a few days in the hospital without them is a good jump start. If you are preparing for scheduled bypass surgery you should strongly consider quitting cigarettes well before the operation to let your lungs and circulatory system begin healing before having to endure the stress of surgery.

To this day, I will sit at a stoplight and watch someone smoking a cigarette and enjoy that. I never mind if people smoke in front of me. It doesn't bother me a bit. I know I've turned the page on that.
Steven S.

Strategies for Quitting

Smoking is a complex addiction. In preparing to quit you need to prepare for both the physical and the psychological withdrawal you'll face. Here are several steps to help you do that:

1. Determine your readiness to quit.
2. Assess your tobacco use.
3. Set a quit date.
4. Determine the best method for quitting.
5. Ask for help.

Find Out If You Are Ready to Quit

I'm not a smoker now, but I was 40 years ago. One day someone showed me a couple of pictures. One was of a pink, healthy lung and the other one was the diseased lung of a smoker. I quit on the spot.
Ivan B.

You can't quit unless you want to. If you feel you aren't ready to quit, make a list of reasons to quit and a list of reasons to continue smoking. Think honestly about your barriers to quitting. Are you afraid of failure? Are you apprehensive about the symptoms of withdrawal? Are you angry about having to change your lifestyle? Addressing these barriers will help you to overcome them.

One physician who was a smoker developed a very logical argument for quitting cigarettes that is worth passing on. He said, in effect, that he would have to quit smoking if he had a heart attack. So why not quit now and avoid the heart attack in the first place? There are other good incentives to stop smoking that are entirely separate from health issues. You will save a lot of money. People won't stare at you in restaurants or ask you to move. You won't have to stand around outside smoke-free office buildings. Your clothes and your hair won't stink.

If you've tried to quit in the past and haven't been able to, don't automatically think you will fail again. There are many resources available to you to help you succeed.

Determine When and Why You Smoke

Every smoker has a different relationship with cigarettes. Find out what yours is by thinking about the number of cigarettes you normally smoke, when you smoke, and under what circumstances. You can better anticipate cravings and avoid personal triggers for smoking if you plan for them in advance.

You can also ask yourself a couple of key questions to determine how physically addicted you are to nicotine.

Do you smoke more than a pack a day? The more cigarettes you smoke each day, the less likely it is that you are smoking because of a behavioral habit or social habit. It is much more likely that you are smoking because your body craves the nicotine. You may want to consider nicotine replacement therapy to help reduce the symptoms of nicotine withdrawal.

Do you smoke more heavily in the morning? When you sleep at night, you are spending 6 to 8 hours without nicotine. If you really crave a cigarette within 30 minutes of waking, or if you smoke several cigarettes in the morning, you are doing so to stave off the symptoms of withdrawal. You may want to change your morning routine in the days before you quit, or add extra coping strategies to deal with this time of day. For example, if you always have a cigarette in bed (which beyond everything else is a bad idea), you may want to get out of bed as soon as you wake up and go read the paper or go for a walk instead. Brush your teeth instead of having the cigarette. Remove the rituals that trigger nicotine cravings in the days before you quit.

How do you feel when you can't smoke? If you have trouble sitting through a movie or a church service without wanting to leave to smoke, or if you smoke when you are bedridden with illness, your addiction is well entrenched. You might consider individual counseling or a support group to help you through the first weeks after you quit. Remember that the more methods you use to quit, the more likely you are to be successful. And if you are a cardiac patient, you have the strongest incentive there is to quit.

Set the Date

When you set a date to stop smoking, give yourself enough time to prepare for the event. Prior to the date, you'll want to remove all ashtrays, cigarettes, and lighters from your home. If you live with a smoker, ask that person to take the habit outside for a few weeks. Your spouse and family members should be eager to help you by not smoking near you. You can talk to family members about specific ways that they can assist. Tell them exactly how their support can boost your confidence in the weeks and months after you quit.

Practice quitting in the days before your quit date. Skip certain cigarettes during the day and try out coping methods to get you through these times. This will give you extra confidence as your quit date approaches.

Dealing with Your Relapses

Many people relapse once or twice before they successfully give up cigarettes. Rather than thinking of a relapse as a failure, look at it as an opportunity to learn how to do better next time. What caused you to slip? Do you need more aggressive methods to cope with your withdrawal?

> *I decided to quit right after my stent was put in. Well, within a week or so afterward. My doctor told me he'd had the best results from patients who used the gum, because it would give you an immediate jolt when you had a craving. It gave me a jolt alright, but that was because it tasted so terrible. In the end, I used the patch—and willpower. That's how I quit three years ago.*
> Oscar M.

Nicotine Replacement Therapy (NRT)

Smokers who are heavily dependent on nicotine have found that using nicotine replacement therapy can ease the symptoms of nicotine withdrawal that make quitting so difficult. NRT comes in several forms such as gum, skin patches, and sprays. In some studies, smokers who use NRT have double or triple the success rates of smokers who don't, but it is the smokers who are most physically addicted to nicotine who benefit the most.

Nicotine gum may be more effective for you than nicotine patches when you first quit. This is because unlike the patch, which provides a stable level of nicotine, gum allows you to tailor the dose of nicotine to your mood in the way you were accustomed to doing with cigarettes. In addition, gum gives you something to open and stick in your mouth, mimicking some of the behaviors you associate with smoking. Maybe it's not pretty, but it can work. Sooner or later you will become tired of using the gum, at which point you may more easily transfer to a brief period of patch replacement before finally stopping.

Precautions for Nicotine Replacement

Some doctors are reluctant to recommend NRT to heart patients, because nicotine in any form will raise your heart rate, but the doses of nicotine given can be lower than those in cigarettes and there is no tar or carbon monoxide, making it safer than continued smoking. A nicotine patch provides from 7 to 21 mg of nicotine over a 24-hour period, while a piece of gum contains from 2 to 4 mg of nicotine.

The nicotine patch has been shown to be relatively safe with some people with heart disease. However, you shouldn't take it if you've had a heart attack within the past two weeks because of the risk of arrhythmias associated with nicotine. For the same reason, patients with serious arrhythmias or unstable angina will probably not be able to take nicotine in any form. Some doctors feel that controlled nicotine replacement is preferable to surreptitious smoking or binge smoking. At least nicotine replacement doesn't reduce oxygen and increase carbon monoxide in the blood as smoking does. Still, nicotine in any form can be dangerous to many heart patients. Be sure to discuss the issue of nicotine replacement with your doctor.

In addition, nicotine patches may not be tolerable for people with severe eczema, an allergy to adhesives, and other skin diseases. Nicotine gum is not advisable for people with jaw problems and for people who wear dentures. Nicotine nasal spray is not advisable for those who have asthma, any infection or inflammation of membranes inside the nose, nasal polyps, or infection inside the sinuses.

Side effects. The patch causes skin irritation, which will require regularly changing the spot where you apply it. Nicotine nasal spray may cause irritation in the nose and throat, watery eyes, sneezing and cough. Nicotine gum can irritate your mouth and gums.

Bupropion (Wellbutrin)

Bupropion was first introduced as an antidepressant in the mid-1980s, but unlike most anti-depressants it has no effect on the brain chemicals serotonin or norepinephrine, or on the enzyme monoamine oxidase. Instead, it may increase the effects of a different neurotransmitter, called dopamine, in the brain. By mimicking some of the pleasurable and relaxing effects of cigarette smoking, it has helped some smokers quit.

What the Research Shows

In one study of 893 patients, 28.8 percent of those taking bupropion had not returned to cigarettes at seven weeks compared to 19.6 percent in the placebo group. After one year, 19.6 percent in the treatment group were still abstinent compared to 12.4 percent in the placebo group. These results seemed to be dose dependent, with people taking higher doses of the drug showing slightly higher success rates. As with any smoking cessation technique, it works best as part of an overall program that includes medical counseling and social support. Because it uses a different mechanism of action than nicotine replacement therapy, it can be used with NRT.

Precautions and side effects. People who have suffered from bulimia or anorexia and those with a seizure disorder should not take bupropion, nor should anyone taking a monoamine oxidase (MAO) inhibitor. Some seizures have been associated with related medications.

Some people experience headache, insomnia, and dry mouth while taking bupropion.

Help Your Spouse to Quit

Your spouse wants to quit smoking, and your help is one of the most important factors in his or her success. Here are some ways you can assist.

State the obvious. People are far more successful at quitting if they believe that it is best for their health. Your spouse is giving up cigarettes in exchange for an improved prognosis. Reinforce this message and let him know that his health is important to you.

Remove temptation. Just before the quit date, help remove the smoking paraphernalia from the house. If you smoke, agree not to smoke in front of him or her and get the help of friends and family in this plan as well.

Be a cheerleader. Praise every milestone. Nicotine withdrawal makes people irritable and short tempered. They sometimes feel depressed, particularly if they begin to gain weight. Offering encouragement and the expectation of success in spite of this irritability is important, and works far better than criticism.

Provide distraction. Identify activities, new and old, that can be enjoyable and perhaps challenging, that can also distract your spouse from thoughts of tobacco.

Get help. The advice and encouragement of a doctor or nurse doubles the success rate of people trying to quit smoking. Even a 5-minute conversation with a doctor or nurse about continuing the effort to quit can have a significant impact on the process.

Some Questions to Ask

Now that you have been diagnosed with heart disease, continuing to smoke will have dire consequences for you. It will elevate your heart rate and blood pressure, while decreasing the oxygen in your system. On the other hand, if you quit smoking, your health can only improve, and that improvement is likely to be dramatic. Most people need help in quitting, and there are several questions you may want to ask yourself or discuss with a spouse or doctor before you quit:

* *Am I ready to quit?*

* *If not, can I make a list of reasons to quit and a list of reasons to continue smoking?*

* *Am I afraid of failure? How can I deal with this fear?*

* *How can my family and friends help me to quit?*

* *Do I need nicotine replacement therapy to help me quit? In what form am I most likely to use it?*

* *What would be an appropriate date to set for quitting?*

* *How can I deal with relapses?*

Chapter 16

✦ ✦ ❖ ✦ ✦ ❖ ✦ ✦ ❖ ✦ ✦ ❖ ✦ ✦ ❖ ✦ ✦ ❖ ✦ ✦

Emotional Risk Factors
The Effects of Stress, Depression, and Anger

The diagnosis of heart disease has an enormous impact on your life, and on your emotional state. A significant number of people with heart disease experience an episode of depression in the wake of a heart attack or surgical procedure. This depression can be mild and may remit spontaneously, or it may be more severe and long-lasting. A chronic depressive state is a powerful negative influence on your health and even on your survival.

Other social and psychological factors in your life, such as chronic stress or hostility, type A behavior and social isolation can also cause or intensify health complications from heart disease. These issues, which doctors call psychosocial factors, can be as important to your health as your lipid levels, your blood pressure, your weight, your sugar control, and your medications.

In this chapter, you'll learn to evaluate your own emotional risk factors and you'll discover how they may be affecting your health. You'll also discover what treatments are available, including talk therapy and medication.

I was a machinist and I had weight restrictions after surgery, so I had trouble with my job. My main worry is financial stuff. That was the problem.

I went in and had bypass surgery, and it didn't take. I went to a different doctor who said that the first bypass wasn't done correctly. The graft wasn't attached far enough away from the clot. The whole surgery needed to be redone. The insurance company doesn't expect to get another bypass in six months, so they refused to pay. And my wife had switched jobs, so it was a pre-existing condition, anyway. So, I'm out of a job, we've got four kids. It was just one financial thing after another. I think we only survived because some people from church brought us dinners and collected cash for us. I guess I'm Mr. Pessimist. I just have a bad outlook. I watched my father die of heart disease after his transplant and it was slow and agonizing.
Lou S.

The Link between Emotions and Health

A cardiac event can cause depression, or it can aggravate a mild depression that you may have been living with for many years. It can certainly trigger anxiety about your health, your job and your finances. All of this can combine to create a fog of gloom and exhaustion that in some cases may seem impenetrable.

Even if it doesn't trigger depression, a cardiac event certainly increases your level of stress, which stimulates the adrenergic nervous system, and in turn increases the work load of the heart. When you are anxious and your heart is pounding, you are at greater risk for heart attack and arrhythmias. If you are a hard-driving perfectionist who is demanding of yourself and others, or if you are someone who often exhibits anger and hostility, your nervous system may already be chronically activated in an adverse way.

Over the past decades, researchers have become increasingly aware of the role of psychosocial factors in patients with heart disease. First, these researchers focused on the dangers of compulsive, time-intense behavior that came to be characterized by Meyer Friedman as the "type A" personality. Later, it was recognized that aggressive and hostile behaviors are associated with cardiac risk. Indeed, studies have shown that a heart attack is far more likely to occur within a couple of hours of a major episode of anger.

More recently, the striking relationship between depression and repeat adverse cardiac events in patients with coronary disease has come under intense scrutiny. It turns out that being depressed or hostile can sharply increase the risk that you'll have another heart attack or stroke, develop a life-threatening arrhythmia, or need another revascularization procedure. Your emotional health also affects the quality of life of your spouse and that of your family. At the same time, your family support system also affects your level of stress.

My husband has been a wonderful father to the children. Now that his angina is so bad, it upsets him to think that he can't do the things he wants to do. His legs ache when he just walks more than a few blocks, so he can't go walking with our kids when they come to visit. One day our son said, "Gee, Dad, you're falling apart." That hurt him for a long time, much more than being housebound. Kids say things, and they don't know how much it can hurt someone who has been active his whole life.
Denise S.

How Widespread Is Depression?

More than 40 percent of heart patients exhibit some signs of clinical depression, particularly in the months following a heart attack. Some researchers put the figure as high as 60 percent. If you have suffered from depression in the past, or if you have been living with heart disease for many years, your risk of experiencing depression in the wake of a coronary event or surgery is especially high. It is important to be aware of the symptoms and to know what treatments are available.

Of course, not everyone is depressed after a cardiac event. Sometimes people who have elective surgical procedures seem to adjust to the event better than people who have emergency or urgent operations or procedures.

When my brother died suddenly, I found out that he had died of a heart attack, even though he was in great shape and had no symptoms of heart disease. I was very upset and anxious about the possibility that I could

*have heart disease, too. I went in for the stress test, and did well. I grad-
ed out at above the 90 th percentile. Given my family history, though, the
doctor suggested a cardiac catheterization and I had that scheduled right
away. Even though they found a blockage and I ultimately had an angioplasty to clear it, I had no emotional response to the procedure at all. It
was like walking into somebody's office for a couple of meetings. It had no
effect on my playing sports, or experiencing pain. A week afterward, I had
almost completely forgotten about it, except that I had to take some pills.
Oscar M.*

When you schedule a cardiac catheterization or even bypass
surgery ahead of time, you have time to ask your doctor questions
about what you will experience. You even have time to organize
your life around the event. But when the need for a procedure
comes with no warning, even the strongest and most confident person may emerge shaken, stunned, and depressed in the recovery
period.

*Right after my surgery, I become so emotional over the smallest things.
Watching TV, those silly stories on TV, and I would get swept away by
them. It could be anything ordinary and I would become emotional. The
doctor had warned me about this. They'd even written it down on some
forms they gave me. So I knew what it was about.
Dennis L.*

What Is Depression?

Depression is a clinical term for a chronic emotional state that interferes with your relationships, your job, and your day-to-day life. This
condition is defined by its characteristics. If you have several of the
following symptoms, you may be depressed.

* *Changes in sleep habits, difficulty falling or staying asleep and waking
  with anxiety, or sleeping many more hours than normal*

* *Changes in eating habits, especially a striking weight gain or weight loss*

* *Difficulty concentrating, remembering things, or making even simple
  decisions*

* *Chronic fatigue or lack of energy, sluggishness*
* *Feeling sad or hopeless*
* *Constant anxiety and fidgetiness*
* *Losing interest in activities and hobbies that you used to enjoy, or with-drawing from family and close friends*
* *Feeling worthless and guilt-ridden, feeling like a failure*
* *Having thoughts of suicide or death*

Remember, everyone has some of these symptoms from time to time. Clinical depression involves more severe and prolonged episodes that interfere with your life.

How Is Depression Diagnosed?

Doctors can diagnose depression using a simple series of questions, or even a questionnaire. It may consist of only two questions or as many as 25 questions that help ascertain your emotional state. The questions themselves are straightforward (Do you often feel sad? Do you have thoughts of suicide?). The doctor will rely on you to answer them honestly. This is no time to pretend that things are well if they are not, which is about as helpful to your health as denying that LDL levels are high or insisting that your blood pressure is normal when it is not.

Like many medical conditions, depression exists on a continuum. You can be mildly, moderately, or severely depressed. Your depression can be temporary, or it can be chronic. Your treatment will be tailored to your symptoms and needs. That is why your honesty is so important.

> *My husband did have depression. Not a bad case of it. He was so quiet, and he wasn't eating. I remember sitting in the waiting room at rehab, where they rest after doing their exercises. This was months after his heart attack and surgery. And I remember someone made a joke, and he laughed and I started to cry. Someone said, "What's wrong?" And I said, "I just heard my husband laugh for the first time since his heart attack."*
> *Lynn K.*

When to Be Concerned

I was having chest pain, so I went to the doctor to get an ECG, and he told me it was angina and sent me home. Four weeks later I had a heart attack. I took a cab to the hospital, but I got stuck in traffic for half an hour. I barely made it into the emergency room before I passed out. I had emergency bypass surgery. Afterward, I had a lot of pain during recovery, and I was a little depressed. I felt, "How could this happen? This is terrible." It was just the shock of it. I was angry at my doctor because I thought he didn't diagnose the problem correctly. I was afraid of dying, and I didn't know when I would get my life back. When would I start running again, which is something I love to do.
Ivan B.

At this point, you may be saying to yourself, "Of course, I'm depressed. I've been hospitalized, I'm in pain, and I'm facing a long recovery." You are partly correct. Having a chronic medical condition can bring on temporary depression.

It's also true that if you go down the list of depression symptoms, you may find that some of them have been caused or exacerbated by your heart attack or the medical intervention used during your treatment. These may include:

Sleeplessness. This is a hallmark of depression. Yet, it is also one of the primary side effects of cardiac surgery. Sleeplessness may be related to lingering effects of anesthesia, sedatives or sleeping pills used in the hospital, or the routine interruptions throughout the night that are common during a hospital stay. At home, the normal healing process often results in extra sleepiness.

Fatigue and lack of energy. Fatigue can be the result of depression, or it can be a lingering side effect of anesthesia, an anemia (reduction in blood cells) that often follows heart surgery, and generalized deconditioning of the body after bed rest. If you have had a major heart attack, some fatigue may be attributable to a reduction in the pumping power of your heart.

Weight loss. In the weeks following a heart attack or surgery weight loss is quite common, and need not be a sign of depression. You may not feel hungry for the foods on your new diet, and you may have a legitimate fear of the junk foods that were once your favorites. Your medications may also be upsetting your stomach.

So it can be difficult to attribute these symptoms to depression with any certainty in the immediate post-event period. As common as these physical side effects are, with progressive healing and medical treatment, they should gradually disappear over the first few weeks of your recovery. If they don't, you could have clinical depression that needs medical attention.

For people with heart disease, the most telling symptoms of depression are:

* *Feelings of hopelessness*
* *Feelings of failure*
* *Finding no pleasure in life*
* *Withdrawal from family and friends*
* *Thoughts of death or suicide*

These are emotional responses that may not directly be related to a heart attack or surgery. They may be signs of depression that are independent of your heart condition. Even if triggered by recent events, depressive symptoms signal an emotional state that can threaten your physical health.

Persistent feelings of hopelessness are particularly dangerous. In fact, these feelings are predictors of future coronary events even in people who have no diagnosis of heart disease. It is not clear why this should be. However, people who feel hopeless about their condition and their future are less likely to take care of themselves, less likely to modify their risk factors, less likely to take prescribed medications, and far less likely to return to the doctor for regular examinations and tests.

Depression Is a Risk Factor

Failure to take care of yourself is not the only side effect of depression. Numerous recent studies have shown that depression increases your risk of dying from heart disease regardless of your other risk factors or even the severity of your condition. One study looked at a group of people with unstable angina and found that those who were also depressed were four times as likely to suffer another heart attack. In another study people suffering severe depression following a heart attack were more than four times as likely as those without depression to suffer a significant decline in health within six months.

People who are depressed also face a longer recovery period after heart attack or surgery. They report more pain than nondepressed people and have more difficulty returning to their normal routine.

One possible reason for this effect is that depression seems to increase episodes of myocardial ischemia in people with coronary disease. Ischemia is the condition in which the heart isn't getting enough oxygen, and it is generally associated with angina.

What the Research Shows

In one study, depressed and nondepressed patients were given mental stress tests and monitored by a portable ECG during their daily activities. Those patients who exhibited mild to moderate depression experienced many more episodes of ischemia than did patients without depression. Being chronically sad seems to place an extra burden on your heart, which can lead to additional damage to the heart muscle and to additional risk of arrhythmias.

Like many risk factors, depression poses a greater threat to your health as its severity becomes more pronounced. Several studies have found that patients suffering from a milder form of depression are at lower risk for cardiac mortality than those with severe depression. Mildly depressed patients are also more likely to respond favorably to treatment.

Social Support Increases Survival

After the first bypass, when he wasn't getting any better, and we went to another doctor to get another catheterization and another opinion, my husband was so scared and depressed. The kids were coming in from other states to visit wondering if they should say good-bye to him, and he was 47. It was pretty frightening. I couldn't deal with it in that way. There was a part of me that needed to be strong, to keep working, to negotiate with bill collectors. I'd heard that attitude is so important. As negative as my husband was, I decided to be that positive.
Denise S.

I'm only alive today because of my wife.
Lou S., husband of Denise S.

During my recovery, my wife never looked so good. When I was flat on my back, she looked more gorgeous than she did on our wedding day.
Donald D.

One factor most likely to improve survival in people recovering from a heart attack is social support. One study followed elderly patients hospitalized for acute myocardial infarction and found that those who had no emotional support were nearly three times as likely to die in the six months following their heart attack than those who had at least one source of emotional support. This was true regardless of the severity of the heart attack, or the number of risk factors the people had for a subsequent heart attack. It was also true regardless of the person's age or gender.

Support did not have to come from a spouse. In fact, people who were unmarried or lived alone but had someone in their lives in whom they could confide or who could occasionally help them with daily tasks had much lower mortality rates than those who were married but reported no emotional support at home. People offer the most important kind of social stimulation, but in some studies, heart patients with pets seem to fare better than those without. The common thread seems to be emotional interaction, which can reduce stress.

Recovery Can Be Spontaneous

Your depression may not be permanent. In fact, it may lift before you can receive medical treatment. For as many as 30 percent of people who show minor signs of depression following a cardiac event, depression is a temporary condition that goes away spontaneously. Doctors refer to this as an adjustment reaction, meaning that you may experience symptoms of depression while you are getting used to your medication, to the new physical sensations and limitations of your condition, and especially to the reality that your life has now changed because of illness.

People who have a history of depression, those who have type A personalities, and those who have no network of family and friends to offer support are the least likely to have their depression disappear on its own. Also, the older you are and the more severe your condition, the less likely you are to have symptoms go away without treatment.

Women and Depression

Women with heart disease are more than twice as likely to be diagnosed as depressed as their male counterparts. This may be because

---

What the Research Shows

One study that seems to support the theory that women are more sensitive to the stress of illness used questionnaires to compare and contrast the reactions of men and women with heart disease. They found that men react primarily to stressors at work, particularly the loss of control, while women react to stressors both at home and at work, particularly those situations in which they feel they have too much to do and aren't getting enough help. Overall, the study showed that women may be more sensitive to the emotional stressors of their condition, and that this emotional sensitivity affects the disease process to a degree similar to other risk factors.

---

women are more inclined to admit to emotional difficulties, or it may be because they tend to be diagnosed with heart disease later in life, at a time when they have fewer resources to help them cope. It may also be because women are more sensitive to the emotional stressors of their illness.

Hostility and Coronary Artery Disease

At rehab, they wanted me to take a written test on anger. I told them it was a stupid test. They wanted to know what I do when people cut me off in traffic. I thought, "Well, sometimes I do nothing, sometimes I shoot the bird and sometimes I'm going to yell out the window." It depends, but they want to pigeonhole me. What's a hostility test, anyway? I told them, "First of all, it's a stupid name for a test." They said, "Well, aren't you being hostile right now?" I said, "Yes, I am. Do I pass?"
Margaret G.

My husband's fear does turn into anger. And then I have to be the negotiator, to make sure people aren't hurt because he lashes out. I sometimes have to phone after and say he's upset and apologize for him. Sometimes I think his anger is so strong that it actually makes him sick.
JoAnne S.

Depression and social stress are not the only emotional risk factors for heart disease. It has long been recognized that type A behavior—defined as unrelenting perfectionism aimed at yourself and those around you—is associated with cardiac risk. So is hostility and cynicism. Studies have shown that people are much more likely to suffer a heart attack within a couple of hours of experiencing a major episode of anger.

Hostility is defined as the need to direct your anger at others, or an inability to control your anger. Cynicism is a belief that others can't be trusted. If you have heart disease, these are dangerous traits. Unlike depression, which can come in bouts, these character traits tend to be consistent and difficult to change.

Hostility, cynicism and type A behavior cause you to overreact to petty frustrations, such as being put on hold, receiving incorrect change from a sales clerk, or hitting all the red lights between home and work. If small inconveniences or frustrations cause you as much emotional turmoil as major crises, then your sympathetic nervous system—the one that triggers the "fight or flight" response—is in a near constant state of activation. While it is activated, your heart rate and blood pressure are elevated, your blood has a tendency to clot, and unstable plaques are more prone to rupture. In the hours following an episode of extreme anger or frustration, you are much more likely to have a heart attack. The more often you experience these moments, the more often you are at risk.

Several studies have closely linked a tendency toward hostility or cynicism with heart disease, fatal heart attack, and the recurrence of arterial blockages after angioplasty and bypass surgery in both men and women. Although hostility and cynicism are most often associated with men, at least one study has looked at their effect on postmenopausal women.

What the Research Shows

In this study researchers interviewed 792 postmenopausal women with coronary artery disease (CAD) and then followed them for a little more than four years. They found that women who were most prone to hostility were twice as likely to suffer a heart attack compared to those at the lowest end of the hostility scale. They were also more likely to have a higher body mass index, higher levels of triglycerides, lower levels of HDL cholesterol, and a worse sense of their own health.

On the other hand, type A people seem to be more compulsively interested in organizing and implementing their treatment, and in seeking medical attention for symptoms. At least one study has indicated that once a type A patient has developed heart disease, he or she tends to manage it more carefully and with better outcome. This part, at least, is a plus.

How Stress Affects Your Body

The important thing to remember about emotional stress is that it takes a physical toll on your body. Strong emotions such as anger and fear activate your sympathetic nervous system, which causes the body to increase production of certain chemicals, called catecholamines (adrenaline is one example). These chemicals affect the body in ways that can have serious consequences for people with heart disease.

For example, catecholamines increase the tendency of your blood to initiate clots. In several studies, researchers have drawn blood from people under chronic job stress and found that their blood was more likely to clot. These chemicals also increase your heart rate and blood pressure which will increase your risk of developing complex and dangerous arrhythmias. Elevated heart rate and blood pressure also make unstable plaques within the arteries more likely to rupture.

The Treatment Paradox

If depression causes an increase in the risk of death from coronary artery disease, it should follow that treating depression, particularly in severely depressed patients, should decrease mortality. Unfortunately, the studies to date have been inconclusive on this point.

Other, smaller studies have shown a significant survival benefit from a wide variety of techniques for treating depression and reducing stress in the wake of a heart attack. Some of these include teaching stress management and relaxation methods as a part of an exercise program or cardiac rehabilitation. Although these studies are not conclusive in terms of improved mortality, they all show that treatment of depression and management of hostility help patients to feel better about their lives. Having a positive outlook is crucial at a time when you will need to take difficult, proactive steps to improve your health.

What the Research Shows

The largest and most recent trial to address this issue was the Enhancing Recovery in Coronary Heart Disease Patients (ENRICHD). In this study, the treatment group received therapy to help decrease social isolation and anxiety, and to help them solve their problems. Severely depressed patients also had the option of taking anti-depressants. Participants in the control group received their usual medical care with no special provisions for therapy or antidepressant medication.

The somewhat surprising result of this study was that patients treated for depression did not have a higher survival rate or fewer heart attacks than those who were not treated. However, patients who received treatment for depression did report improved social support and quality of life. The smaller subset of patients who actually took antidepressants to treat their depression were at lower risk for another heart attack or death. By the end of the study 20 percent of the control group patients along with 28 percent of the treatment group were taking antidepressants to treat their depression.

Treatment Reduces Your Healthcare Costs

Treating depression may seem to be just another bill to pay, more appointments to keep, and more pills to take. However, without treatment, your depression will probably add more to your health care costs than therapy ever will.

What the Research Shows

One study followed 848 survivors of acute myocardial infarction and tracked their health care costs through Medicare in Canada. Those patients with severe depression cost the Medicare system an average of 41 percent more in total costs than patients without depression. These costs stemmed from longer stays in the hospital, more emergency room visits, and more visits to doctors other than cardiologists.

The study's findings suggest that because your emotional health impacts the amount of money you spend on health care every year, improving that aspect of your health is a good investment.

Available Treatments

A number of options are available to help you feel better emotionally. These include talk therapy, regular exercise, antidepressant medication, and antianxiety medication. If you join a cardiac rehabilitation program, you may have the chance to learn about other methods, including relaxation, stress reduction, and techniques for identifying and reducing type A behavior. Many patients choose their own combination of therapies from any or all of these options.

> *My husband has been in group therapy. It's a support group for cardiac patients. He doesn't like being the youngest guy there by several years. He keeps bucking it. It's a great challenge to get him to stay in the room for three minutes, but he's doing it. I think it helps him to be able to hear other people talking about what they're going through, even if he doesn't like talking about his own feelings.*
> *Denise S.*

Goals of Talk Therapy

Therapy is more than just an opportunity to talk to someone about yourself and your problems. It is the chance to really be heard at a time when your family and friends may not be able to listen appropriately or may not know how to respond. Psychotherapy does not have to stretch on for years and years. You can decide along with your therapist whether you need it to last a few weeks or a few months. This type of therapy is agenda-based, meaning that you and your therapist will have specific, stated goals, including:

* *Getting you involved again in the activities and relationships that were once so important to you*

* *Actively solving your problems, or finding new strategies to help you cope with your life*

* *Talking frankly about the negative thoughts and habits that serve as stumbling blocks in your relationships*

* *Developing positive strategies such as ways to reinforce healthy self-esteem*

Choosing a Therapist

When you decide to seek counseling, you are looking for someone to help you improve your life—or at least your ability to cope with your problems. You'll want to choose someone who has worked with cardiac patients before, someone who is familiar with the issues you are likely to face, including stress at home, limitations at work, and even the financial burden of illness. A therapist who regularly works with cardiac patients will be familiar with the medications you are taking, and will know about a range of social services available to help you if you need them.

This person might be a psychiatrist (a medical doctor trained in dealing with emotional issues), a clinical psychologist, a social worker, or sometimes a religious counselor. You may want to choose someone recommended by your cardiologist or who is affiliated with the hospital or practice where you received treatment.

It is important that you and your therapist agree to keep in mind all three aspects of your condition—the mental, the environmental, and the biological. Being in treatment with a therapist who comes from a background similar to your own and is likely to share your values works best. Finally, you don't have to love your therapist, but if he or she does not command your faith and respect, feel free to look somewhere else.

Antidepressants

My husband doesn't think his antidepressant does anything, but it does. We all notice the difference. He took it for a while and then when he quit, I didn't know what I was going to do. His mood is so black, and his energy is so low without it. I kept encouraging him to go back on it, and so were the nurses who work with his cardiologist. Finally, we wore him down. He said, just get me the damn prescription. I ran back to the nursing station and said, "Now. Now. Give it to him now."
Dana M.

A decade ago, antidepressants were considered to carry some risks for heart patients. The two most common types of drugs prescribed to depressed patients, monoamine oxidase inhibitors (MAO inhibitors) and tricyclic antidepressants, had effects on the cardiovascular system that were often undesirable for patients with heart disease. These drugs sometimes increased heart rate, and could bring on abnormal heart rhythms, and rarely, heart block. In addition, they sometimes caused orthostatic hypotension, a condition in which the blood pressure drops suddenly as you get out of bed in the morning or rise from a chair.

Fortunately, a newer group of antidepressants, called selective seratonin reuptake inhibitors (SSRIs), have come along in the past decade. These include fluoxetine (Prozac), sertraline (Zoloft), paroxetine (Paxil), citalopram (Celexa), escitalopram (Lexapro), Fluvoxamine (Luvox), and venlafaxine (Effexor). These drugs have fewer side effects and seem generally safe for heart patients. They also seem to have very few drug-food interactions or drug-drug interactions, which makes them safer for patients already taking several medications. However, their use should be carefully monitored. Bupropion (Wellbutrin) is not an SSRI but it can be used to treat depression and to help with smoking cessation. Low doses (25 to 50 mg at bedtime) of trazedone (Desyrel) can be used to enable sleep.

How they work. The nerve cells of the brain communicate with each other by releasing chemical substances, called neurotransmitters into the space between one nerve ending and the next nerve cell. This space is called a synapse. After a neurotransmitter has been released into the synapse, it is then absorbed by the nerve cell. There are quite a few chemicals that operate in this manner in the brain, and one of them is called serotonin. It seems to regulate both mood and appetite. Low serotonin levels in the brain have been associated with depression, and drugs that increase the serotonin effect in the brain can improve mood and reverse serious depression.

The effect of a neurotransmitter depends on how much of it is released and how long it remains active in the synapse between cells. The faster the neurotransmitter is taken up by the nerve ending that released it, the less its effect will be. Conversely, the slower its absorption, or reuptake, the greater its effect.

Selective serotonin reuptake inhibitors (SSRIs) are drugs that reduce the removal of serotonin that is released into the synapse. By blocking reuptake into the nerve ending, the chemical effect of serotonin present in the synapse is increased. The result is a natural lift in mood and a suppression of appetite. Sometimes these drugs also reduce anxiety. SSRIs do not have marked effects on other neurotransmitters, but other antidepressant drugs with less selective modification of synapses may block reuptake of norepinephrine and dopamine as well as serotonin. Individual responses to these different drugs will vary, and sometimes the best response requires a combination of medications under careful medical supervision.

Dosing. Your doctor may begin with a low dose of a particular SSRI and then see how well you tolerate it for a few days before increasing the dose. It may take several attempts to find the dose that works well for you. These drugs take anywhere from four to six weeks to exert their full effect, so while you may experience an earlier improvement, you should not conclude that the drug isn't working until a sufficient amount of time has elapsed.

The improvement produced by these drugs is often subtle and gradual, not dramatic like taking a tranquilizer of some sort. It is also important not to stop taking them without conferring with your doctor. You may need to take them for six to eight months, or even longer.

Precautions and side effects. These drugs have far fewer side effects than older antidepressant medications. However, some people notice mild side effects, particularly in the early weeks of taking them while your doctor may be adjusting the dosage. Be sure to talk to your doctor about any symptoms you think may be related to your medication. As a heart patient, you are probably taking several medications already. Because interaction of drugs can produce complications, it is important to discuss these potential effects with your physician. This is particularly true for a class of drugs called monoamine oxidase inhibitors, a group of antidepressants that should not be mixed with other drugs without careful supervision.

Guidelines for Your Family

The night before my husband's second bypass surgery, one of our kids called the hospital to tell me that the younger one was really swollen. I drove home and it was true. Our younger son looked like he had the mumps. I packed them both in the car to take them back to the hospital, to the emergency room and that's when I slammed the car door on my hand. My hand was broken, my wedding ring was smashed and we still had to get to the hospital. When we walked in the door, I said to the admitting nurse, "My insurance card is in my pocket, but you're going to have to get it out, and my husband is having surgery upstairs and he can't know any of this." I knew as a spouse that whatever I was going through, it had to take a backseat to his surgery. It all worked out, and my husband never knew anything about it until the surgery was over.
Denise S.

Everyone's concerned about the person who's had the heart attack, but there's another person who's walking a parallel track. And it's OK for someone to say how are you doing? And the answer is you're scared absolutely out of your wits.
Lynn K.

As the spouse or close family member of a heart patient, you are in a unique position to observe the emotional changes of your loved one. Unfortunately, you may also bear the brunt of the sadness, bitterness, and anxiety as it arises in your spouse. Your support and help are a crucial component in your spouse's recovery. Numerous studies have shown that mildly depressed patients are more likely to respond to treatment and to recover if they feel loved and supported by family and friends.

Similar studies have also shown that this is not true of people who are severely depressed. They are likely to be unresponsive to your efforts to care for them. They may even be hostile to your care, so you will need outside additional help.

Sometimes you need a break. In Miami when he quit smoking he was a bear. And I said, "Why are you mean to me, and you're not mean to the

nurses?" And he said, "They'll quit on me if I yell at them." I said, "Well, guess what, I'm quitting." And I walked out. I heard him calling after me, but the nurses outside his room gave me the thumb's up. I came back in a few minutes, but I'd made my point.
Dana M.

If you are living with someone who is severely depressed, you are probably familiar with these negative attitudes:

Catastrophic thinking. Looking at everything as black or white.

Discounting positives. Feeling that milestones in recovery, such as an uneventful stress test or low cholesterol reading, don't matter.

Magnification of the negative. Feeling certain that the worst will always happen.

Selective sabotage. Picking out a single negative detail to focus on in every situation.

Sweeping generalizations. Making disparaging pronouncements about the motives of others or the way the world works.

Caring for someone with a serious medical condition can be exhausting. Trying to buoy his or her spirits as well can be impossible. Not only can it leave you physically and emotionally drained, it can put your health at risk. Remember that your ability to treat your spouse's emotional problems is as limited as your ability to cure his or her physical condition. If you have offered emotional support, and it has been rejected, speak with your spouse's cardiologist about treating his or her depression with medication or therapy.

By now, you are probably familiar with your role as a patient advocate, someone who asks questions of medical professionals to clarify the diagnosis and the treatment options available, and someone who demands quality medical care when it seems lacking. Now, you will likely have to take on the new role of medical advocate, someone who urges the patient to seek treatment for depression or hostility or uncontrolled anxiety. Heart patients suffering from depression often insist that they are not really depressed. They may also view depression as a weakness, and in light of their new physical limitations, having to admit to an emotional weakness as well may be unbearable. Convincing a spouse or family member to see a therapist or to speak with a doctor about depression may take some time.

Taking your own meds is so hard. You forget to have them with you in case you stay overnight in the hospital. That's when friends and family can be so helpful. They can walk your dog. They can bring your meds to the hospital, or some pajamas. There were times when I drove home over an hour to take the dog out and then back to the hospital in the middle of the night and that's dangerous. I remember being mad at people for not helping me, when I'd never asked for help. I think people would have done anything for me if I'd asked.
Denise S.

The first one to two weeks at home after bypass surgery were a veritable nightmare. I could hardly lift my legs or stand up. Fortunately, Medicare provided a nurse to check my medical status, and a wonderful home aide who helped me bathe and dress. I also had a rehabilitation specialist who gave me progressive exercises to regain my strength. Those three professionals provided important support for my family, too.
Frank F.

Remember, it is important for you to take care of yourself both physically and emotionally. Accept help from others when you can, and reach out to your friends when you need assistance or someone to talk to.

Some Questions to Ask

The diagnosis of heart disease can have a lasting effect on your emotional well-being. Many people experience episodes of depression in the wake of a heart attack, angioplasty or bypass surgery. This depression may be mild or it may remit spontaneously. If it does not, if it becomes severe enough to interfere with your ability to function, you should talk to your family as well as your doctor about possible treatment options. Some questions you might ask are:

* *Could my lingering physical symptoms such as sleeplessness, fatigue, and weight loss be a sign of depression?*

* *If so, what are my treatment options?*

* *Who can I reach out to for emotional support?*

* *Could therapy help me cope with my problems?*

* *If so, what does therapy cost? Is it covered by insurance?*

* *Am I a good candidate for anti-depressant medication?*

* *What does medication cost?*

* *What are the side effects of anti-depressants? Can this medication interfere with other drugs I'm currently taking?*

Afterword

by Frederic Flach, MD, KCHS

♦ ♦ ❖ ♦ ♦ ❖ ♦ ♦ ❖ ♦ ♦ ❖ ♦ ♦ ❖ ♦ ♦ ❖ ♦ ♦

I felt particularly enthusiastic about the opportunity to write a brief afterword to this invaluable book. Not only have I spent decades investigating the nature and treatment of clinical depression, but I have also personally benefited from the marvels of modern cardiovascular medicine. I have long believed that an important connection existed between untreated depression and cardiovascular disease, and this premise has finally been established through careful research.

Early in my medical career, there were few meaningful treatments for a heart attack. Patients, if they survived, were hospitalized for about six weeks for rest and observation. Often, they had to make major lifestyle changes. They were encouraged to rest often, reduce physical activities, perhaps retire from work, and regard themselves as invalids. Since consequent congestive heart failure was a frequent occurrence and could be treated primarily only with diuretics to rid the body of excess fluid, a salt-free diet, and digitalis to strengthen heart muscle, life expectancy was limited. Controlling blood pressure was a profound challenge, since none of our contemporary anti-hypertension drugs were available. As recently as 1965, about 40 years ago, my own father died suddenly of heart disease at the age of 75. Had he been born 15 years later, his lifespan might have been extended another decade or more.

My own brush with cardiac illness began very much by happenstance. I had been in good health, with no symptoms suggesting circulatory problems. I had a history of modestly elevated blood pressure, but this had been well managed with medication for years. I had been a smoker in the past. Most World War II veterans were, since in those days, nobody associated smoking with cancer or heart disease. Besides, during the war, most of us were more concerned about staying alive another few days or months, not another 50 years.

For a number of years, I worked out three times weekly with a trainer. I was able to lift 170 pounds on the leg press machine and 80 pounds on the weight pulley. I have never been overweight, averaging 172 pounds on my 6-foot, 1-inch frame. I seldom ate fatty foods, although I did enjoy a good steak and beef ribs now and then. My cholesterol—both the HDL and LDL—were well within normal limits. However, I may have had more than my fair share of stress in my lifetime, including a condition called post-traumatic stress disorder (PTSD) since my early twenties.

In the spring of 2000 I came down with a viral endocarditis (inflammation of the lining of the heart) and pleurisy (inflammation of the lining of the lung). These afflictions were extremely painful. I had little appetite and lost seven or eight pounds. But after a few weeks I felt better and resumed my normal activities, seeing patients, writing, editing a medical journal, and running a continuing education program for medical professionals. In April 2001, I volunteered to have a spiral CAT scan. It was quite a new procedure at the time. I had read about it in the bulletin of New York Presbyterian Hospital, where I'm on the attending staff.

The results were a profound shock. The normal level of calcium that should be detected in the coronary arteries with this test is several hundred milligrams. My reading was in the thousands, indicating the need for further tests. An echocardiogram and a thallium stress test were suspicious but inconclusive. So, one bright, sunny morning a few weeks later I found myself slightly sedated but still awake, lying on an operating table at the hospital. A long tube with a small camera at its end was running painlessly up a main artery to my coronary arteries, while the doctors watched its progress on a black and white screen. When the examination was nearly done, I asked my colleagues, "Do I go home now, or do I have an angioplasty and go home tomorrow?"

Their answer was completely unexpected. "You're nearly 90 percent obstructed. Tomorrow morning you must have bypass surgery."

I accepted the news calmly. Fortunately, I've been blessed with a good deal of spiritual faith, and I felt secure in God's good will, whatever the outcome. Of course, I was determined to do my best to survive and recover.

In the hospital, I was well looked after. I still had the anesthetist's intubation tube in my throat when I awoke in the intensive care unit, but I had been warned that I would not be able to speak until it was removed. I had a blackboard to write on, although I wasn't inclined to write very much on it. My family was allowed to visit right away, adding to my sense of warmth and security.

A day or two later—I don't actually recall, since the passage of time in a hospital is often a blur—I was transferred out of the ICU to a regular unit. There, I was immediately encouraged to become active and walk. So I walked, and walked, and walked, unsteadily at first, but gaining strength and confidence with each attempt.

Then I was discharged and I could not have anticipated the turmoil that was to follow. I was taken downstairs in a wheelchair. I needed help to get in the car, to struggle out of it when we reached home, and even to lift my feet to put them up on an ottoman. I felt a kind of weakness I never recall having felt before in my life. Medicare paid for a nurse to come twice a week to check my pulse and blood pressure and other relevant signs; a physical therapist three times a week to assist me with my exercises; and a home health aid to help me with bathing and dressing. I was really an invalid. And I felt like an invalid as I slowly walked along the corridor of our apartment house, lifting one heavy foot in front of the other and stopping periodically to regain my breath.

Somewhere around my third week back home I began to feel depressed. On one level I felt I was going to be fine. On another, I felt old, sad, irritable, with a sort of "what's the point of it all" attitude. Luckily, and thanks in part to my religious faith, this mood cleared up in a week or so, and by July I was actively engaged in a full-fledged cardiac rehab program such as the one described in this book.

In many ways, I think this period was tougher on my family than on myself. They were terrified that I might die, and watching someone who is normally strong and vibrant become so debilitated must have been a profoundly disturbing sight. They indeed rallied to my side, my wife, children, and pastor, hour-by-hour, day-by-day, others with their phone calls and prayers. I must have received more than 100 get-well and prayer cards.

I had a few other medical issues to deal with that complicated my recovery, including a close call in the fall of 2001. Because of the pleurisy I had had the year before, the surgeons could not use the mammary artery as one of the major bypass grafts. So they had to use a vein instead. Unfortunately, veins are not as strong as arteries. The one supplying the major part of my heart collapsed. A large part of my heart "went to sleep" and stopped functioning due to a lack of blood supply. The doctors refer to this phenomenon as hibernation. As a result, I suffered mild congestive heart failure. Fortunately, however, there was no significant damage to the heart muscle and a difficult but successful angioplasty with stents was done.

In the winter of 2002 I went through cardiac rehab again, and it played a pivotal part in my recovery. I have resumed my regular trips to the gym, although I don't engage in quite as strenuous exercises as before. Now, more than two years later, I must say I feel like a young man much of the time.

I am one of the fortunate ones. I did not have a heart attack, and thus my heart muscle has not been significantly damaged. Had the diagnosis of advanced coronary arteriosclerosis not been made serendipitously, I'd have been a candidate for suddenly dropping dead—in a crowd of nameless faces, in the middle of dinner with friends, on the beach on some remote Caribbean island. But now I can look ahead to a number of happy and productive years to come.

There was that brief time, right after surgery, when I didn't feel so hopeful. I was depressed. But I knew enough to expect it. On the other hand, a close fried who underwent bypass surgery a few months after I did was caught by surprise; he became very distressed to find himself crying uncontrollably and prudently called me for reassurance. Actually, depression is quite common following cardiac surgery, and perfectly normal if it resolves itself in a few weeks or less. However, patients whose down moods hang on are not only more likely to have trouble recovering from heart attacks, but they are also more prone to die from them. Moreover, recent studies clearly demonstrate that chronically depressed men and women are more likely to develop cardiovascular illness in the first place. This puts undiagnosed and/or untreated depression up there as a significant risk factor for heart disease, along with elevated cholesterol, high blood pressure, smoking, obesity, and lack of exercise.

The cardiac rehab program is an excellent setting in which to present the facts about depression and refer those patients who qualify for this diagnosis to appropriate professionals for treatment. More broadly, primary care physicians and cardiologists should be alerted to this risk and prepared to regularly assess all their patients for depression and see that they get care they need.

This is easier said than done. There is still a stigma attached to the idea of being depressed. People still consider it a "mental illness," a character weakness, or a lack of spiritual fiber. Health professionals are no exception. There is still a lot of confusion and consternation about what depression really is. Is it a normal human experience? When does it become an illness? Is it primarily physical? Can it be effectively treated?

In my book, *The Secret Strength of Depression*, now in its 3rd Revised Edition, I described a new way to view depression, one that has helped alleviate stigma and has proved helpful to patients and professionals alike. I have found that patients more readily accept the idea of being depressed and take steps to seek treatment when the following formulation is offered to them.

There are many times and situations in which depression is a normal and healthy reaction. It becomes a medical issue when it is too extreme and/or when the depressed person cannot bounce back on his or her own in a reasonable period of time. Then it's called *chronic* depression, persisting for months, even years, and continuing to be a disabling and disruptive force in one's life.

The factors responsible for this misfortune have more to do with a *lack of resilience* than with depression itself. They fall into three categories. The first is psychological and pertains to personality traits and behaviors that affect how well or poorly you handle stress and change.

The second is physical, involving hormonal and other chemical events within your body, especially within your brain, which have to do with thought processes, emotions, and behavior under a wide variety of circumstances. When these aren't operating as they should, it can be hard, if not impossible, to pull out of a depressed mood. . . and this is where antidepressant medications come in. It's always important to rule out specific illnesses too, such as hypothyroidism, which may be adding to the problem.

Finally, the conditions surrounding you can help or hinder recovery, a loving family as opposed to a hostile spouse, good working conditions versus horrific ones or long-term unemployment complete with financial desperation.

Why is chronic depression a risk factor for heart disease? We have few clues. Certain behaviors, like smoking and lack of exercise, are more common in depressed people. Years ago, my colleagues and I discovered that chronically depressed patients pulled calcium out of bone, depositing it in soft tissues and also excreting it from the body in large amounts. With successful treatment using antidepressant medications, this flow was reversed and calcium was again laid down in bone. Could such calcium changes contribute to a loss of elasticity in blood vessels, thus creating a better climate for the deposit of fatty plaques and eventual obstruction of blood flow? Or does the heart disease-behavioral connection involve inflammatory processes, the immune system, or something else as yet unsuspected?

For the time being, these ideas remain in the realm of speculation. What is no longer speculative is that rehabilitation for the cardiac patient that includes appropriate medications, lifestyle changes such as diet, exercise, and freedom from nicotine, as well as the treatment of clinical depression and efforts to strengthen resilience can make a dramatic difference as far as patients' outcome and longevity, and the quality of their lives.

—*Frederic Flach, MD, KCHS*
Attending Psychiatrist, New York Presbyterian Hospital
Attending Psychiatrist, St. Vincent's Hospital and Medical Center,
New York

Appendix I

◆ ◆ ❖ ◆ ◆ ◆ ❖ ◆ ◆ ◆ ❖ ◆ ◆ ◆ ❖ ◆ ◆ ◆ ❖ ◆ ◆ ◆ ❖ ◆ ◆

Commonly Used Cardiovascular Medications

[Adapted from 2003 Physicians Desk Reference with additions]

Peripheral Adrenergic Blockers

Aldomet (Methyldopa)
Apresoline (Hydralazine)
Cardura (Doxazosin)
Hytrin (Terazosin)
Minipress (Prazosin)

Combined Alpha and Beta Adrenergic Blockers

Coreg (Carvedilol)
Normodyne (Labetalol)

Angiotensin Converting Enzyme (ACE) Inhibitors

Accupril (Quinapril)
Altace (Ramipril)
Capoten (Captopril)
Lotensin (Benazepril)
Monopril (Fosinopril)
Prinivil (Lisinopril)
Vasotec (Enalapril)
Zestril (Lisinopril)

Angiotensin II Receptor Blockers (ARBs)

Atacand (Candesartan)
Avapro (Irbesartan)
Benicar (Olmesartan)
Cozaar (Losartan)
Diovan (Valsartan)
Micardis (Telmisartan)

Beta-Adrenergic Blocking Agents (Beta-Blockers)

Blocadren (Timolol)
Corgard (Nadolol)
Inderal (Propranolol)
Kerlone (Betaxolol)
Lopressor (Metoprolol tartrate
a short acting form of metoprolol)

Sectral (Acebutolol)
Tenormin (Atenolol)
Toprol-XL (Metoprolol
succinate, a long acting
form of metoprolol)
Visken (Pindolol)
Zebeta (Bisoprolol)

Bile Acid Sequestrants

Colestid (Colestipol)
Questran (Cholestyramine)
Welchol (Cholsevelam)

Fibric Acid Derivatives

Lopid (Gemfibrozil)
Tricor (Fenofibrate)

HMG-CoA Reductase Inhibitors (Statins)

Crestor (Rosuvastatin)
Lescol (Fluvastatin)
Lipitor (Atorvastatin)
Mevacor (Lovastatin)
Pravachol (Pravastatin)
Zocor (Simvastatin)

Calcium Channel Blocking Agents

Adalat (Nifedipine, in a
   shorter acting form)
Adalat CC (Nifedipine, in a
   sustained release form)
Cardizem (Diltiazem, in a
   shorter acting form)
Cardizem SR (Diltiazem, in a
   sustained release form)

Loop Diuretics

Demadex (Torsemide)
Edecrin (Ethacrynic acid)
Lasix (Furosemide)

Potassium-Sparing Diuretics

DynaCirc (Isradipine)
Isoptin SR (Verapamil, in a
   sustained release form)
Norvasc (Amlodipine)
Plendil (Felodipine)

Aldactone (Spironolactone)
Dyrenium (Triamterene)
Midamor (Amiloride)

Thiazide and Related Diuretics

Procardia (Nifedipine, in a
shorter acting form)
Procardia XL (Nifedipine, in a
sustained release form)
Tiazac (Diltiazem, in a
sustained release form)
Verelan (Verapamil, in a
sustained release form)

Diuril (Chlorothiazide)
HydroDiuril
(Hydrochlorothiazide)
Lozol (Indapamide)
Microzide
(Hydrochlorothiazide)
Renese (Polythiazide)
Zaroxolyn (Metolazone)

Antiplatelet and Anticlotting Agents

Aspirin
Clopidogrel (Plavix)
Ticlid (Ticlopidine)
Warfarin (Coumadin)

Combination Diuretics

Aldactazide (Spironolactone
plus Hydrochlorothiazide)
Dyazide (Triamterene plus
Hydrochlorothizide)
Hyzaar (Losartan plus
Hydrochlorothiazide)
Lotensin HCT (Benazepril plus
Hydrochlorothiazide)
Maxzide (Triamterene plus
Hydrochlorothiazide)
Moduretic (Amiloride plus
Hydrochlorothiazide)

Coronary Vasodilators

Isordil (Isosorbide dinitrate, medium duration)
Nitro-Dur (Nitroglycerin in a sustained release transdermal skin patch)
Nitrostat (Nitroglycerin tablets for sublingual use, rapid acting)
Imdur (Isosorbide mononitrate, long acting)
Ismo (Isosorbide mononitrate, long acting

Appendix II

◆ ❖ ◆ ❖ ◆ ❖ ◆ ❖ ◆ ❖ ◆ ❖ ◆ ❖ ◆ ❖ ◆ ❖ ◆

Glossary

Adrenaline: Also known as epinephrine, this is a catecholamine released from the adrenal glands that stimulates the body's "fight or flight" response.

Amino acids: Organic compounds that link to form proteins. The body needs about 20 different amino acids to function normally. Some of these amino acids, known appropriately as "essential amino acids," cannot be manufactured by the body and must therefore be obtained from food. *See also* Protein.

Anemia: A reduction of the number of red blood cells, which can reduce the amount of oxygen transported in the blood stream.

Aneurysm: A bulge in an artery that weakens the arterial wall and may cause it to burst or bleed.

Angina: Chest discomfort caused by a temporary imbalance between the heart's demand for oxygen and its supply. The discomfort is often described as a pressure in the center of the chest that may extend to the left arm or to the back or to the neck, or sometimes just as a sense of shortness of breath. It is usually brought on by exercise or emotional upset and relieved by rest. Angina ordinarily occurs with incomplete obstruction of one or more of the coronary arteries that supply oxygen to the heart. *See also* Stable Angina and Unstable Angina.

Angioedema: An allergic condition in which patches of tissues swell. This can be a rare allergic reaction to ACE inhibitors that prevents some people from taking these drugs.

Angiogram: An X-ray picture of the blood flow in an artery or vein, created by using a catheter to inject a liquid into the lumen (inside) of a blood vessel that blocks transmission of X-rays. This allows doctors to visualize the location and severity of obstructions in these vessels, ultimately creating a road map for defining and treating them. *See also* Cardiac Catheterization.

Angiography: The process of obtaining an angiogram.

Angioplasty: A catheterization treatment to open an artery that is blocked by an atherosclerotic obstruction. It is performed by inflating a balloon at the end of a specialized catheter inside the obstruction, and it is sometimes followed by placing a stent at the site of angioplasty.

Angiotensin: A chemical that causes constriction of arteries throughout the body, which produces increased pressure and greater resistance to blood flow. More precisely known as Angiotensin II, it is formed from a precursor chemical called Angiotensin I by the action of angiotensin converting enzyme.

Angiotensin Converting Enzyme (ACE): A substance that promotes the production of angiotensin (Angiotensin II) in the body.

Angiotensin Converting Enzyme (ACE) Inhibitor: A class of drugs that reduces the production of angiotensin by reducing the effect of angiotensin converting enzyme. These drugs tend to lower blood pressure and the resistance to blood flow by reducing the constriction of arteries.

Angiotensin Receptor Blockers (ARBs): A group of drugs that block the effect of angiotensin by directly blocking the receptors in the arteries that react to angiotensin.

Anticoagulants: A drug designed to prevent blood clots in both arteries and in veins by suppressing the production of an enzyme called thrombin.

Antiplatelet Medications: A group of drugs that reduce the stickiness of platelets and reduce the release of substances from platelets that promote blood clots at the site of injury or inflammation inside arteries.

Aorta: The main artery leading from the left ventricle to the body that delivers oxygen rich blood through the large systemic arteries to the major organs.

Aortic Valve: The valve leading from the left ventricle to the aorta that keeps blood from flowing backwards into the heart from the aorta.

Arrhythmia: An irregularity of the normal rhythm of the heart. These include simple extra beats, groups of extra beats, rhythms that are too slow or too fast. Most arrhythmias of the heart are not immediately dangerous, but some serious arrhythmias can lead to shock or cardiac arrest.

Atherosclerosis: A disease of arteries in which plaques composed of fat and fibrous tissue accumulate within the inner lining of the vessel. These atherosclerotic plaques may become large enough to obstruct or occlude the artery.

Atrial Fibrillation: A common type of arrhythmia in which irregular rapid electrical activity in the atria causes ineffective contraction in the atria. Even so, the ventricles continue to pump relatively normally, although irregularly. A major problem associated with atrial fibrillation is the potential formation of blood clots in the noncontracting atrium. These clots may escape from the heart to cause a stroke or other blockage of an important artery in the body.

Atrium: The two upper chambers of the heart, connecting to the ventricles. The right atrium receives unoxygenated blood from the veins in the body and empties through the tricuspid valve into the right ventricle, which pumps blood through the pulmonic valve into the pulmonary artery of the lung. The left atrium receives oxygenated blood from the lungs and empties into the left ventricle, which pumps blood through the aortic valve into the aorta.

Automatic Implantable Cardioverter-Defibrillator (AICD): a device designed to monitor each heartbeat, like a regular pacemaker, but capable of delivering a shock to the heart to restore a normal heart rhythm and therefore to treat potentially fatal arrhythmias, such as ventricular tachycardia and ventricular fibrillation. Some of these devices also function as pacemakers, and some have separate modes of treatment for different heart rhythms. *See also* Defibrillator.

Autonomic Nervous System: The part of the nervous system that regulates involuntary responses of the body, that is, those that do not require or depend on conscious control. It consists of the sympathetic nervous system, which prepares you for wakefulness and the "fight or flight" response, and the parasympathetic nervous system, which prepares you for relaxation and sleep.

Azotemia: An accumulation of waste products in the blood due to decreased kidney function.

Beta-Adrenergic Blockers: A class of drugs that block the stimulation of the beta-receptors of the body. In the heart, beta-blockers reduce the heart rate and the force of contraction of heart muscle to reduce the overall workload of the ventricles. These drugs are a cornerstone in the treatment of heart attacks because they can decrease the damage to heart muscle and decrease the chances that the heart will suffer a fatal arrhythmia. They are also a cornerstone in the treatment of angina and they can be valuable in the treatment of some patients with hypertension.

Bile Acid Sequestrants: A type of medication that binds up the cholesterol-rich bile acids in the small intestines to prevent their reabsorption into the body. This has the effect of lowering the amount of cholesterol in the system.

Biventricular Pacemaker: Uses synchronized pacing of the heart by two separate wires, one to each ventricle, to better simulate the heart's normal electrical activity.

Body Mass Index (BMI): A calculation of body weight adjusted for height. The formula for calculating your BMI is weight in kilograms divided by height in meters squared.

Brachial Artery: The artery in your upper arm. This is usually the artery in which your blood pressure is measured.

Bradycardia: An abnormally slow heart rate. Certain medications can exacerbate this condition.

Bradykinin: A chemical that stimulates the relaxation of arteries, which increases blood flow.

Brionchioles: The tiny tubes that bring air from the larger bronchi into the tissues of the lungs where oxygen can be extracted.

Bupriopion: An antidepressant medication that has sometimes been effective in helping smokers quit.

Bypass surgery: Also known as coronary artery bypass grafting surgery (CABG). This is a major operation in which blood flow is routed around clogged coronary arteries. The detour can be constructed using veins or arteries that are attached to the aorta and to the coronary artery, or an internal mammary artery can be rerouted to the obstructed coronary artery. Bypass surgery generally involves opening the chest and use of a heart-lung machine, but occasionally the surgery can be performed through a limited incision on the beating heart.

Calcium Channel Blockers: A group of medications that reduce the flow of calcium ions from the blood into heart muscle cells or into the smooth muscle cells that cause constriction of the blood vessels. These drugs can lower blood pressure by reducing resistance in the arteries, and some can reduce the contraction power of the heart. Calcium blockers are sometimes used to control the heart rate in atrial fibrillation.

Capillaries: The smallest component of the circulatory system, these tiny vessels lead from the smallest arteries to the smallest veins to supply blood directly to the tissues and organs of the body.

Carbohydrate: A chemical energy source in food that is composed of carbon atoms combined with hydrogen and oxygen in the proportion found in water. This large class of chemicals includes sugars, starches, and cellulose.

Cardiac Arrest: A fatal condition in which the heart fails to pump effectively. The most common cause of cardiac arrest is ventricular fibrillation, a rapid and disorganized electrical activity of the ventricles, but cardiac arrest can also occur if the electrical activity of the heart stops entirely. Cardiac arrest is the main cause of death in the period immediately following a heart attack.

Cardiac Catheterization: A technique for inserting small tubes, called catheters, through the arteries and veins into the heart. Catheters can measure the pressures in the chambers of the heart and can be used to transmit x-ray blocking liquids into the heart chambers and the main arteries of the body, including the coronary arteries. This process, called angiography, allows x-ray pictures of the shape of the heart chambers and blood vessels to be taken.

Cardiac Ischemia: A state of metabolic abnormality in the heart that is caused by an imbalance in the energy (blood and oxygen) supply and demand. Cardiac ischemia may cause chest discomfort and weakness of the heart. During temporary ischemia (such as angina), the heart muscle may normalize at the end of the event, but when ischemia is prolonged (as in a heart attack), the heart muscle may be permanently injured.

Cardiac Output: The amount of blood pumped into the circulation, as measured in liters per minute. This is a measure of the overall performance of the heart.

Cardiac Rehabilitation: A formal program of exercise training and risk factor education designed to help heart patients improve confidence, effort capacity, and lower cardiac risk.

Cardiologist: A specialist in the care of patients with diseases of the heart and circulatory system.

Cardiopulmonary resuscitation (CPR): A procedure developed in the late 1950s to provide a measure of effective circulation during cardiac arrest by mechanically compressing and relaxing pressure on the heart through the chest wall while providing artificial respiration.

Cartoid Arteries: Two large arteries in the neck that supply blood to the brain.

Catecholamines: A group of chemicals secreted by the adrenal glands and present in some nerve endings that prepare the body for stress. These include epinephrine (also known as adrenaline), and norepinephrine and dopamine.

Catheterization: The process of inserting small tubes called catheters into the body, especially into blood vessels. *See also* Cardiac Catheterization.

Cholesterol: A structural fat used by the body to maintain the membranes of individual cells, to waterproof the skin, to promote digestion, and to build the body's hormones.

Cilia: The hairs in cells that line the small airways inside the lungs and help to remove mucus and debris.

Circulatory Shock: A condition in which blood flow is so low that the major organs of the body cannot function normally. This results from limited oxygen delivery and a build-up of waste products in the cells.

Claudication: Pain, cramping, or muscle weakness in the muscles of the legs that generally occurs with exercise and is relieved by rest. It is caused by atherosclerosis in the arteries that feed these muscles, and it usually is a sign that atherosclerosis is quite advanced. Claudication of the leg muscles is analogous to angina in the heart, since both are due to temporary and reversivle limitation of blood supply. If limited blood supply to the limb becomes so severe that prolonged ischemic injury causes death of the skin or muscle tissue, gangrene may occur. Gangrene in a limb is analagous to myocardial infarction in the heart, with damage that is no longer reversible.

Clot-Busting Drugs: A group of drugs, such as streptokinase and tissue plasminogen activator (TPA), that can dissolve blood clots that have already formed inside arteries. These drugs are used in the treatment of acute heart attacks and can be important in limiting the damage done by other arterial blockages, such as those that cause some forms of stroke.

Coronary Arteries: The blood supply to the heart muscle. There are three major coronary arteries. Two of these, the left anterior descending (LAD) artery and the left circumflex artery, branch from the large left main (LM) coronary artery that originates in the aorta, while a third, the right coronary artery, originates directly from the aorta.

Coronary Artery Bypass Grafting Surgery (CABG): *See* Bypass Surgery.

Coronary Care Unit: A hospital unit designed in the 1960s to care exclusively for cardiac patients, particularly patients with heart attacks.

Coronary Spasm: An abnormal contraction of part of a coronary artery that can reduce blood flow to the heart muscle, a relatively rare cause of angina or, when spasm is sustained, of a heart attack.

C-Reactive Protein (CRP): A chemical produced by the liver in the presence of infection of chronic inflammation in the body.

Cyclo-Oxygenase: An enzyme that stimulates the production of thromboxane in platelets and prostacylin in the endothelial cells of the arteries. Thromboxane promotes blood clots, while prostacyclin relaxes the arteries. Aspirin is an inhibitor of cyclo-oxygenase that in lower doses reduces the production of thromboxane more than that of prostacyclin.

Defibrillator: A machine developed in the 1950s to deliver a DC current shock the heart to restart it after cardiac arrest due to ventricular fibrillation. Early defibrillators were so large and heavy that patients at risk were clustered in coronary care units to be near them. Now, defibrillators the size of small pacemakers can be implanted in individuals.

Diabetic Retinopathy: An affection of the blood vessels of the eye that can produce blindness in people with diabetes.

Diastolic Blood Pressure: The bottom number of the fraction that expresses your blood pressure reading. This is the the pressure in your arteries between heart beats, during relaxation of the heart.

Diuretics: Drugs that lower blood pressure by lowering salt, water and blood volume in the body.

Drug eluting stents: Stents that have been coated with medication to reduce the production of scar tissue around the stent. These stents slowly release their drug coating into the artery to prevent smooth muscle cells and scar tissue from building up around the stent.

Echocardiogram: A non-invasive procedure in which a two-dimensional picture of the beating heart is obtained by reflection of sound waves from the chest. It is used to measure the size of the chambers of the heart, to assess heart function and to examine the heart valves, among other things.

Edema: Extrusion of fluid from the blood into the body tissues by high pressures in the circulatory system. Swelling of the extremities, particularly of the legs, can result from high venous pressures and is called peripheral edema. Fluid in the lungs as a result of high pressures in the heart is called pulmonary edema. Edema is a common symptom of heart failure from a number of different causes.

Efferent Arteriole: A second set of arterioles after the glomerulus in the kidney that plays a role in setting the filtering pressure in the glomerulus.

Ejection Fraction: The proportion of blood present at the beginning of contraction that the left ventricle expels with each beat. In a healthy heart this is likely to be 50 to 70 percent, because not all blood is squeezed out with each cycle. Ejection fractions below 40 percent are usually due to generalized or to localized heart muscle damage.

Electrocardiogram (ECG, also known as EKG): A non-invasive recording of the heart's electrical activity. Often used to diagnose damage from a heart attack or rhythm irregularities, and may be observed during exercise testing.

Electrolytes: Minerals, including potassium, sodium, chloride, and magnesium, that the body requires for proper function of the cells. Some medications, such as diuretics, can upset the balance of these chemicals, causing muscle weakness, dizziness and other problems.

Endothelial Cells: The cells that line the inside of the arteries.

Epinephrine (adrenaline): *See* Adrenaline.

Fat: Fats are chemical substances that contain three fatty acid chains attached to a glycerol molecule; for this reason they are known as triglycerides. Each of the fatty acid chains is composed of a series of carbon atoms that are capable of bonding with hydrogen. These carbon bonds can be completely saturated, polyunsaturated or monounsaturated with respect to hydrogen atoms.

Fibric Acids (Fibrates): These drugs decrease the production of very low density lipoprotein (VLDL) triglycerides and help to metabolize triglycerides.

Fibrillation: A condition in which the electrical activity in a heart chamber becomes disorganized, leading to disorganized contraction. *See also* Atrial Fibrillation, Ventricular Fibrillation.

Foam Cells: Macrophages that have ingested oxidized LDL in the arterial endothelium.

Framingham Heart Study: One of the early landmark population studies of the evaluation of risk for heart disease and the prediction of its complications, which began in 1948 and continues to this day in Massachusetts.

Glomerulus: The filtering unit of the kidneys.

Glucose: Blood sugar, a simple and common carbohydrate.

Glycemic Index: a measure of how fast and far your blood sugar level goes up after eating a particular food. Complex carbohydrates such as beans and whole grains tend to have a "lower glycemic" index than simpler carbohydrates such as processed sugars.

Glycosylated Hemoglobin (HbA1C): A measurement that reflects the average sugar level of the blood over several weeks to months.

Heart Block: A type of arrhythmia caused by an inability of the heart's natural electrical impulses to reach the pumping chambers of the heart.

Heart Failure: A chronic, progressive condition in which the heart can no longer effectively pump adequate amounts of blood.

Heart-Lung Bypass Machine: A machine that performs all the functions of the heart and lungs, keeping oxygenated blood moving through the body while the heart is temporarily stopped during surgery.

Heart Rate: The number of cardiac contractions per minute.

Heart Rate Recovery: How quickly your heart rate returns to normal after exercise. This rate of recovery is likely to be lower among heart patients and deconditioned people, but it can increase as you increase your level of fitness.

Hemoglobin: A protein in red blood cells that carries oxygen molecules through the blood stream.

Hemorrhagic Stroke: Damage to the brain from a burst blood vessel.

High Density Lipoprotein (HDL): Also known as "good cholesterol," these lipoproteins are thought to carry LDL away from the arteries to be eliminated as waste by the liver. A high level of HDL particles has a protective effect against heart disease.

Homocysteine: An amino acid. High levels of homocysteine in the blood have been associated with blood clots and the accelerated accumulation of arterial plaque. May also be related to high stress and vitamin deficiencies, especially of folic acid and vitamin B12.

Hyperkalemia: An abnormal build-up of potassium in the blood, which can be related to a number of conditions such as kidney failure, diabetes, and shock, and to some medications.

Hypertension: High blood pressure, that is, blood pressure readings above 130/85.

Hypertrophy: An adaptive process by which muscle tissue becomes thicker and stronger when it works harder. Hypertrophy of the heart means an increase in total mass of the heart and takes several forms. Concentric hypertrophy refers to the thickening and stiffening of the wall of the heart that occurs when the heart's ventricle struggles to pump blood against high pressure in the arteries. Eccentric hypertrophy occurs when the heart becomes larger by dilating.

Hypoglycemia: Critically low blood sugar, which may be associated with confusion, sweating, and rapid heart beating.

Hypoperfusion: A condition in which blood flow to the tissues is not adequate for normal function. This is the effect of heart failure on the body.

Hypotension: Abnormally low blood pressure that can result in episodes of dizziness and lightheadedness, especially when getting up from a seated or reclining position. Certain medications can cause or exacerbate this condition.

Implantable Cardioverter-Defibrillator (ICD): *See* Automatic Implantable Cardioverter-Defibrillator.

Implantable Pacemaker-Defibrillator: *See* Automatic Implantable Cardioverter-Defibrillator.

Infarcted Area: The area of damaged cells in the heart muscle after a heart attack.

Infarction: Prolonged ischemia that leads to death of cells in the affected tissue or organ. *See also* Myocardial Infarction, Ischemic Stroke.

International Normalized Ratio (INR): A standardized measurement of the effect of the anticoagulant drug warfarin that is used to regulate dosing of the drug. It is more reproducible among different laboratories than the older Prothrombin Time test alone.

Insulin Resistance: A condition in which the cells of the body do not react properly to insulin, making them less able to efficiently use the sugar energy in the foods you eat. This results in elevated blood sugar levels that can lead to d iabetes.

Ischemia: A condition in which the blood supply to an organ does not match the demand of the tissue for oxygen and blood flow adequate for normal function. It can be caused by a reduction of blood supply, or to an increase in blood demand by the organ. The injury caused by ischemia is not necessarily permanent if the blood supply-demand balance is restored before infarction occurs.

Ischemic Stroke: Damage to the brain caused by a limitation of blood supply caused by atherosclerotic arteries to the head. Stroke is to the brain as heart attack (myocardial infarction) is to the heart.

Left Anterior Descending Artery: A coronary artery that provides blood to the front and the sides of the left ventricle as well as the wall of muscle tissue that divides the two ventricles.

Left Ventricular Dysfunction: This is a condition in which the left ventricle, the heart's main pumping chamber, isn't pumping blood as efficiently as it should because of systolic or diastolic functional abnormalities. *See also* Heart Failure.

Leptin: a protein that seems to play a role in the regulation of appetite and energy metabolism. An inadequate amount of this may cause obesity.

Lipoproteins: Molecules of various sizes that carry cholesterol and triglycerides through the body. *See also* High Density Lipoprotein, Low Density Lipoprotein.

Lipoprotein (a): A type of fat particle that seems to be avidly attracted to developing atherosclerotic plaques. It may turn out to be a risk factor of even greater importance than LDL in some people.

Loop Diuretics: A generally more powerful type of diuretic, or water pill, than the traditional thiazide-type diuretics.

Low Density Lipoprotein (LDL): Also known as "bad cholesterol," these particles bring fat to the endothelial cells of arteries during the development of atherosclerosis. A high level of these particles is associated with the progression of heart disease, while lowering of these levels by diet, exercise, and drugs can reduce cardiac events and stroke.

Macrophages: A type of white blood cell that responds to toxins or infection inside the body. These cells ingest oxidized LDL in the arterial wall to become "Foam Cells" that promote growth of the atherosclerotic plaque.

Mammary Artery: A branch of the subclavian artery that can be separated from the chest wall and directly used to bypass obstructions in a coronary artery.

Maximal Heart Rate: The highest rate at which your heart will beat during exercise.

Meta-analysis: A statistical overview study in which the data from several studies are pooled into one larger group to increase the likelihood of determining significant effects.

Metabolic Syndrome: A cluster of findings associated with an increased risk of atherosclerotic heart disease. Markers for this condition include low levels of HDL cholesterol, high levels of triglycerides, abdominal obesity, high blood pressure and high blood sugar levels.

Mitral Valve: The valve leading from the left atrium to the left ventricle that keeps blood from returning to the atrium during ventricular contraction.

Monounsaturated Fat: A type of fat in which only one carbon bond is not combined with hydrogen. This type of fat tends to lower total cholesterol and LDL or "bad" cholesterol and may even raise HDL or "good" cholesterol levels.

Myocardial Cells: The cells that make up the heart muscle.

Myocardial Infarction: This is known commonly as a heart attack. It is caused by a blockage in a coronary artery that is severe enough and prolonged enough to cause death of some of the heart muscle cells. The most common cause of myocardial infarction is a rupture of an unstable coronary artery plaque in patients with atherosclerosis, which produces a cascade of clotting events that may begin with the sticking of platelets to the site of rupture.

Myocardial Ischemia: An imbalance of oxygen supply and oxygen demand in the heart. If not prolonged, and there is no heart muscle damage, reversible myocardial ischemia generally causes angina. When this imbalance is prolonged and cannot reverse itself, it produces myocardial infarction (a heart attack). *See also* Angina, Myocardial Infarction.

Myocardial Rupture: This is a tear in the wall of the ventricle that has become weakened and soft early in the course of myocardial infarction. It may be fatal.

Myoglobin: A protein that combines with oxygen within the muscle fiber and increases the diffusion of oxygen throughout the muscle fiber.

National Heart Lung and Blood Institute (NHLBI): A U.S. government branch of the National Institutes of Health that focuses on research in cardiovascular diseases.

Nephron: One functional unit of the kidney, containing arteries, glomeruli, and tubules. Each one of these 1 million units filters blood and removes toxins from the blood to form urine.

Nicotine Replacement Therapy (NRT): A group of medications, either in patch, spray or gum form, which supply nicotine (but without tar or smoke) to reduce the effects of withdrawal for heavy smokers who are trying to quit.

Nicotonic Acid (Niacin): This is a B vitamin (Vitamin B3). In high doses it helps to reduce LDL cholesterol and increase HDL cholesterol levels.

Nitrates: A group of medications that act as vasodilators by increasing nitric oxide to decrease the resistance in arteries and veins. In addition to increasing flow in coronary arteries, these drugs can decrease the oxygen demand of the working heart.

Nitric Oxide: A chemical produced in the body that dilates arteries; this is the "relaxing factor" present in endothelium.

Nitroglycerin: A rapidly acting medication, generally dissolved in pill form under the tongue, that can increase nitric oxide levels to dilate arteries. Nitroglycerin works like the nitrates, but with faster onset and shorter duration of action. It can also be given intravenously. *See also* Nitrates.

Norepinephrine: A chemical similar to epinephrine (adrenaline) that is released from the adrenal gland and also by the body's sympathetic nervous system during times of stress or physical activity. This substance constricts various arteries in the body and raises blood pressure.

Nutritionist: A dietician who can help create a meal plan that fits your particular health requirements.

Occluded: Blocked.

Off-Pump Coronary Bypass: CABG performed on a beating heart, with a less invasive incision and a smaller scar, but this procedure is usually only performed on patients in the lowest risk groups. *See also* Bypass Surgery.

Omega-3 Fatty Acids: A type of monounsaturated fat that actually helps to lower total cholesterol levels. This fat is found in cold-water fish and in some nuts.

Orthostatic Hypotension: A condition of dizziness in which the blood pressure drops for a time just after you get out of bed in the morning or when you rise rapidly from a chair. It can be worsened by some medications.

Pacemaker: An implanted device designed to intermittently or permanently replace the heart's natural electrical current to regulate the heart rhythm.

Parasympathetic Nervous System: Part of the autonomic nervous system, which regulates your involuntary responses to the world. This component prepares you for relaxation and sleep. *See also* Autonomic Nervous System, Sympathetic Nervous System.

Percutaneous Transluminal Coronary Angioplasty (PTCA): The long term for angioplasty.

Peripheral Arterial Disease: Atherosclerotic plaque that blocks the arterial blood supply to organs other than the heart and brain. Major areas of involvment include the kidneys, digestive organs, and the major muscles of the legs. A common symptom of peripheral atherosclerosis is exercise-related leg muscle cramps.

Plaque: The expression of atherosclerosis in the wall of arteries. Plaque begins as a fatty streak in the artery and progressively enlarges with incorporation of inflammatory type cells that lead to accumulation of fat and fibrous tissue.

Plaque Rupture: A tear in an atherosclerotic plaque that often stimulates the platelets in the blood to initiate a blood clot. This is the most common cause of myocardial infarction. *See also* Myocardial Infarction.

Platelets: A specific type of blood cell that initiates blood clotting at a site of endothelial injury, particularly in the arteries.

Polyunsaturated Fat: These are fats in which two or more carbon atoms are not combined with hydrogen. These fats tend to lower total cholesterol levels and the LDL or "bad" cholesterol levels in your blood.

Potassium: A mineral used by the body's muscles, including the heart muscle in order to function properly. Some medications can affect the amount of potassium in the body. *See also* Hyperkalemia.

Pre-eclampsia: Critically high blood pressure that develops late in pregnancy.

Primary Prevention: Identifying and altering risk factors in people without evident heart disorders to prevent or to delay the development of heart disease. See also Secondary Prevention.

Prostacycline: A potent vasodilator of the prostaglandin class, found in endothelium.

Protein: A complex organic compound composed of chains of amino acids, sometimes called "the building blocks of life." Proteins form many of the structural and necessary chemical elements of life.

Prothrombin Time: A blood test to determine how quickly the blood clots. It is especially useful for people taking anticoagulant medications that interfere with the blood's ability to clot. *See also* International Normalized Ratio.

Pulmonic Valve: The valve leading from the right ventricle to the pulmonary artery that keeps blood from flowing backward into the heart from the pulmonary artery.

Pulse Pressure: The difference between the systolic and diastolic blood pressures. A high pulse pressure is also called isolated systolic hypertension.

Reinfarction: Suffering a second heart attack.

Relative Risk: The risk of having an outcome event, such as a heart attack or stroke, based on one or more risk factors compared with not having those risk factors.

Renal-Adrenal System: Includes the kidneys and the adrenal glands. This system modulates your blood pressure.

Renal Arteries: These supply arterial blood to the kidneys.

Renin: A chemical excreted by the kidneys into the blood that causes a precursor protein to form angiotensin I, which in turn is converted to angiotensin II (generally known simply as angiotensin) by angiotensin converting enzyme.

Renin-Angiotensin System: Includes the effects and internal regulation of both renin and angiotensin.

Resistant Hypertension: A type of high blood pressure that does not easily come into control even with several blood pressure medications.

Restenosis: Closure of an artery at the site of prior angioplasty or stent implantation. Within days, this may be due to blood clots, but later on it may be due to the growth of scar tissue and infiltration of muscle cells at the site. It rarely can produce an even worse obstruction than existed before the procedure.

Resting Heart Rate: The heart rate when the body is at rest. The usual resting rate in normal people ranges from 50 to 90 beats per minute and can be slower in well conditioned subjects. Heart rate rises with exercise, fever, anemia, thyroid disease, and many other problems.

Revascularization: The interventional process of restoring blood flow to blocked arteries on an elective or emergency basis. Methods of revasclarization include angioplasty, stenting and bypass surgery.

Rhabdomyolysis: A rare condition in which skeletal muscle cells break down and release toxins into the blood stream. This condition can be caused or exacerbated by certain medications, including the statin drugs.

Risk Factors: These are findings that have been associated with or directly contribute to cardiovascular disease. These include heredity, age and sex, smoking, high cholesterol, high blood sugar, sedentary lifestyle, hypertension, and stress.

Salt-sensitive Hypertension: A type of high blood pressure that is sensitive to the volume increase in blood plasma that occurs with increased salt intake.

Saturated Fat: A type of fat, usually a solid, in which all the carbon atoms are combined with hydrogen. These fats tend to raise cholesterol levels in the blood and are not good for you.

Secondary Prevention: Taking steps to reduce your risk factors for suffering a heart attack or stroke after you have been diagnosed with heart disease. *See also* Primary Prevention.

Selective Serotonin Reuptake Inhibitors (SSRIs): A type of antidepressant that blocks serotinin reabsorption by nerve endings in the brain, therefore boosting localized serotonin levels along with mood. These drugs have fewer side effects for heart patients than older generations of antidepressants.

Septum: The wall of muscle tissue that divides the two ventricles in the heart. It normally pumps in coordination with the left ventricle.

Serotonin: One of the chemicals released by platelets during the initiation of the blood clotting process. Serotonin causes small arterioles to constrict and reduce blood flow to the blood vessel.

Serum Cardiac Markers: Substances released into the blood stream during a heart attack. These include Creatine Kinase-MB, Cardiac-specific Troponin T, and Troponin I.

Skeletal Muscles: The working muscles of the body, attached to bones.

Smooth Muscle Cells: The contractile muscles in internal organs, including the blood vessels. These cells in the arterial wall regulate constriction and relaxation of the artery.

Stable Angina: Angina whose characteristics are predictable and unchanging in terms of the amount of exercise or emotional distress that leads to symptoms, with a relatively constant frequency of symptomatic events. The implication is that there are no major underlying changes or instability of obstructive plaques. *See also* Angina.

Stable Plaque: Atherosclerotic plaques that are less likely to rupture, either because of less fat, less inflammation, or less mechanical stress. *See also* Unstable Plaque.

Statin: A class of drugs designed to lower the level of cholesterol in the blood stream. These drugs are also administered during a heart attack to help stabilize coronary plaque.

ST Depression: An abnormal finding on an electrocardiogram (ECG) that suggests that some of the heart muscle cells are ischemic.

ST Elevation: An abnormal finding on an electrocardiogram that suggests not only that some heart muscle cells are ischemic, but that a heart attack may be in progress.

Stent: A tiny mesh tube placed in the artery at the site of the blockage after angioplasty to help prevent the artery from closing up. Some stents contain drugs that reduce the likelihood of restenosis.

Stroke: An ischemic injury to the brain that causes death of brain cells, with resulting neurologic damage.

Stroke Volume: The amount of blood ejected by the left ventricle of the heart during each heart beat.

Sulfonylureas: A type of medication that stimulates the production of insulin as a way of treating type 2 diabetes.

Sympathetic Nervous System: The part of the autonomic nervous system that controls automatic responses to stimuli that require alertness and action. This stimulation is also called the "fight-or-flight" response. It prepares the body for confrontation and response to trauma.

Systolic Blood Pressure: The top number of the fraction that represents your blood pressure. This is the pressure against the large artery walls during each heartbeat when the heart is ejecting blood from the ventricle into the arterial system.

Tachycardia: Rapid heart rate.

Thallium Scan: A non-invasive imaging procedure that examines the uniformity of injected thallium uptake by the cells of the heart. Because thallium uptake is dependent on blood flow, it can indicate areas of inadequate or limited flow during exercise caused by coronary disease. Since uptake also requires active myocardial cells, these scans taken at rest can also indicate areas that have suffered prior myocardial infarction.

Thiazide Diuretics: Some of the most widely-prescribed medications for high blood pressure. Also called a water pill.

Thiazolidinediones: A type of medication that increases the body's sensitivity to insulin as a way of treating type 2 diabetes.

Thrombin: An enzyme used by the blood's defense system to create blood clots. This enzyme gathers up bits of fibrous protein to seal a blood clot over the internal wound.

Thrombosis: A blood clot.

Thromboxane A2: A substance released by blood platelets at the site of an internal injury to stimulate the blood clotting system. It stimulates other platelets to stick together to form a temporary plug over the injury site.

Trans-Fatty Acids: A type of unsaturated fat that is unhealthy. Found in margarine, partially hydrogenated vegetable oil and snack foods such as potato chips, this fat tends to raise total cholesterol levels.

Transient Ischemic Attack (TIA): A temporary shortage of oxygen to the brain. If the lack of oxygen becomes critical and prolonged, it may cause a stroke. A TIA is to stroke as angina is to a heart attack.

Tricuspid Valve: The valve leading from the right atrium to the right ventricle that keeps blood from returning to the atrium during ventricular contraction.

Triglycerides: The major form in which fat is stored for release into the bloodstream as a source of energy.

Type A Personality: Compulsive, time-intense behavior that can adversely affect your health.

Unstable or Crescendo Angina: Episodes of angina that are becoming more severe or more frequent, or are precipitated by less and less exercise. In contrast to stable angina, the implication here is that coronary atherosclerotic plaque is changing its composition, size, or stability. *See also* Angina.

Unstable Plaque: Atherosclerotic deposits with a high proportion of fat and inflammatory cells that are more prone to rupture under stress than stable plaques.

Variant Angina: A fairly rare type of angina caused by a spasm in the coronary arteries that reduces blood flow to the heart muscle.

Vascular System: The blood vessels of the body, including arteries and their branches, capillaries, and veins and their branches.

Vasodilators: Drugs or chemicals that dilate the blood vessels.

Ventricles: The major pumping chambers of the heart. The left ventricle pumps oxygenated blood through the aortic valve to the body via the aorta, while the right ventricle pumps de-oxygenated blood through the pulmonic valve to the lungs.

Ventricular Fibrillation: Irregular rapid electrical activation of the ventricle with disorganized contraction of individual heart muscle cells. This is fatal, because the pumping of the heart stops.

Ventricular Remodeling: Enlargement, thickening, or dilatation of the ventricle as a result of having suffered damage during a heart attack.

Vertebral Arteries: Arteries in the back of the neck that supply blood to the central areas of the brain.

Warfarin: An anticoagulant medication that helps prevent the formation of blood clots.

White Coat Hypertension: A tendency in some people to become nervous while their blood pressure is being taken, which causes an inappropriately high measurement, which is temporary.

Appendix III

◆ ◆ ❖ ◆ ◆ ◆ ❖ ◆ ◆ ◆ ❖ ◆ ◆ ◆ ❖ ◆ ◆ ◆ ❖ ◆ ◆

Resources

Organizations and Government Agencies

American Heart Association
www.americanheart.org
1-800-AHA-USA-1
1-800-242-8721
The American Heart Association is a national voluntary health agency whose mission is to reduce disability and death from cardiovascular diseases and stroke. The association has recently begun a new program that offers a free "Learn and Live Quiz" to help users learn more about their heart health. The quiz, which takes only a couple of minutes to complete, is available free by calling 1-888-AHA-CARES or logging on to www.americanheart.org.

Clinical Trials
www.clinicaltrials.gov
A service to patients from the National Institutes of Health (NIH) and the National Library of Medicine (NLM), this site tracks the results of important clinical research and can be searched according to type of disease.

National Heart, Lung, and Blood Institute (NHLBI)
www.nhlbi.nih.gov
301-592-8573
An information clearinghouse for patients suffering from heart, lung, and blood disorders, a division of the National Institutes of Health (NIH).

On-Line Resources

HeartCenterOnline, Inc.
www.heartcenteronline.com
The mission of the HeartCenterOnline is to be the premier cardiovascular specialized health care site on the Internet, to provide cardiovascular patients, their familie,s and other site visitors with the tools they need to better understand the complex nature of heart-related conditions, treatments, and preventive care, and to provide services and applications that deliver value to cardiovascular practices.

MedlinePlus
http://medlineplus.gov
On-line information from the world's largest medical library, the National Library of Medicine. MedlinePlus has extensive information from the National Institutes of Health and other trusted sources on over 650 diseases and conditions. There are also lists of hospitals and physicians, a medical encyclopedia and a medical dictionary, health information in Spanish, extensive

information on prescription and nonprescription drugs, health information from the media, and links to thousands of clinical trials.

Support Groups
Mended Hearts
7272 Greenville Avenue
Dallas, TX 75231
(800) HEART99
www.mendedhearts.org
A national nonprofit organization affiliated with the American Heart Association. Mended Hearts partners with 460 hospitals and rehabilitation clinics and offers services to heart patients through visiting programs, support group meetings and educational forums.

Recommended Reading

American Heart Association, *The American Heart Association Quick & Easy Cookbook: More Than 200 Healthful Recipes You Can Make in Minutes.* (New York: Clarkson Potter, 2001).

Berkson, B., and Challem, J., *Syndrome X: The Complete Nutritional Program to Prevent & Reverse Insulin Resistance.* (John Wiley & Sons, 2001).

The Cornell Illustrated Encyclopedia of Health: The Definitive Home Medical Reference. Edited by Antonio M. Gotto. Weill Cornell Health Ser. (Washington D.C.: Lifeline Press, 2002).

Flach, A., *Combat Fat.* (New York: Hatherleigh Press, 2003).

The National Institute of Aging, *Fitness over Fifty.* (New York: Hatherleigh Press, 2003).

Flach, F., MD, KCHS, *Resilience.* (New York: Hatherleigh Press, 1997).

Flach, F., MD, KCHS, *The Secret Strength of Depression.* (New York: Hatherleigh Press, 2004).

Farquhar, J. W., and Spiller, G., PhD, *Diagnosis: Heart Disease.* (New York: Norton, 2001).

Gersh, B. J., *The Mayo Clinic Heart Book.* (New York: William Morrow, 2000).

Ornish, Dean. *Dr. Dean Ornish's Program for Reversing Heart Disease: The Only System Scientifically Proven to Reverse Heart Disease Without Drugs or Surgery.* (New York: Random House, 1990).

Pashkow, F.J., and Liboy, C., *The Women's Heart Book.* (New York: Hyperion Press, 2001).

Pritikin, Nathan. *The Pritikin Program for Diet and Exercise.* (New York: Bantam Books, 1983).

Yale University School of Medicine Heart Book. Edited/Illustrated by Barry L. Zaret, et al. (New York: Hearst Books, 1992).

Appendix IV

◆ ❖ ◆ ❖ ◆ ❖ ◆ ❖ ◆ ❖ ◆ ❖ ◆ ❖ ◆ ❖ ◆ ◆

Selected Bibliography

Ades et al. "Skeletal muscle and cardiovascular adaptations to exercise conditioning in older coronary patients." Circulation. 1996; 94: 323-30.

Alexander. "Obesity and Coronary Heart Disease." *American Journal of the Medical Sciences*. April 2001; 321: 215-224.

Berkman et al., "Emotional Support and Survival after Myocardial Infarction." *Annals of Internal Medicine*. Dec. 15, 1992; 117: 1003–8.

Berman et al., "The Effect of Aggressive Lowering of Low-Density Lipoprotein Cholesterol Levels and Low-Dose Anticoagulation on Obstructive Changes in Saphenous Vein Coronary Artery Bypass Grafts." *New England Journal of Medicine*. Jan. 16, 1997; 336: 153-62.

Bondestam et al., "Effects of Early Rehabilitation on Consumption of Medical Care During the First Year after Acute Myocardial Infarction in Patients >=65 Years of Age." *American Journal of Cardiology*. 1995; 75: 767-771.

Brotons et al., "Obesity, Cinderella of CHD Risk Factors." *European Heart Journal*. May 2000; 21: 793-5.

Burg et al., "Depression in Chronic Medical Illness: The Case of Coronary Heart Disease." *JCLP/In Session*. Nov. 2001; 57(11): 1323-37.

Chaput et al., "Hostility Predicts Recurrent Events Among Postmenopausal Women with Coronary Heart Disease." *American Journal of Epidemiology*. 2002; 156: 1092-99.

Chobanian AV, Bakris GL, Black HR, Cushman WC, Green LA, Izzo JL Jr, Jones DW, Materson BJ, Oparil S, Wright JT Jr, Roccella EJ; National Heart, Lung, and Blood Institute Joint National Committee on Prevention, Detection, Evaluation, and Treatment of High Blood Pressure; National High Blood Pressure Education Program Coordinating Committee. "The Seventh Report of the Joint National Committee on Prevention, Detection, Evaluation, and Treatment of High Blood Pressure: The JNC 7 Report." *JAMA*. 2003; 289: 2560-72.

Daly et al., "Long-Term Effect on Mortality of Stopping Smoking after Unstable Angina and Myocardial infarction." *British Medical Journal*. July 30, 1983; 287: 324-6.

Detry et al., "Increased Arteriovenous Oxygen Difference after Physical Training in Coronary Heart Disease." *Circulation*. July 1971; 44:109-118.

Ehsani et al., "Improvement of Left Ventricular Contractile Function by Exercise Training in Patients with Coronary Artery Disease." *Circulation*. Aug. 1986; 74: 350-358.

Enos, et al., "Coronary Disease Among United States Soldiers Killed in Action in Korea." *Journal of the American Medical Association*. July 18, 1953; 152: 1090-1093.

Expert Panel on Detection, Evaluation, and Treatment of High Blood Cholesterol in Adults, "Executive Summary of the Third Report of the National Cholesterol Education Program (NCEP) Expert Panel on Detection Evaluation and Treatment of High Blood Cholesterol in Adults (Adult Treatment Panel III)." *Journal of the American Medical Association.* May 16, 2001; 285: 2486-2497.

Frasure-Smith et al., "Depression and Health-Care Costs During the First Year Following Myocardial Infarction." *Journal of Psychosomatic Research.* 2000; 48:471-8.

Friedberg, CK., *Diseases of the Heart*, 3rd ed. (Philadelphia and London: W.B. Saunders, 1966).

Giannuzzi et al., "Attenuation of Unfavorable Remodeling by Exercise Training in Postinfarction Patients with Left Ventricular Dysfunction." *Circulation.* 1997; 96: 1790-97.

Gibbons et al., "ACC/AHA 2002 guideline update for the management of patients with chronic stable angina: a report of the American College of Cardiology/American Heart Association Task Force on Practice Guidelines", 2002. Available at www.acc.org/clinical/guidelines/stable/stable.pdf.

Gruberg et al., "The Impact of Obesity on the Short-Term and Long-Term Outcomes after Percutaneous Coronary Intervention: The Obesity Paradox." *Journal of the American College of Cardiology.* Feb. 20, 2002; 39:578-84.

Hallman et al., "Psychosocial Risk Factors for Coronary Heart Disease, their Importance Compared with Other Risk Factors and Gender Differences in Sensitivity." *Journal of Cardiovascular Risk.* 2001; 8: 39-49.

Hennekins, C. "Aspirin and the Treatment and Prevention of Cardiovascular Disease." *Annual Review of Public Health.* 1997; 18: 37-49.

Herlitz et al., "Smoking Habits in Consecutive Patients with Acute Myocardial Infarction: Prognosis in Relation to Other Risk Indicators and to Whether or not they Quit Smoking." *Cardiology.* 1995; 86: 496-502.

Hoit et al., "Influence of Obesity on Morbidity and Mortality after Acute Myocardial Infarction." *American Heart Journal.* Dec. 1987; 114: 1334-41.

Hurlen, et al., "Warfarin, Aspirin, or Both after Myocardial Infarction." *New England Journal of Medicine.* Sept. 26, 2002; 347: 969-74.

Jiang et al., Depression and Increased Myocardial Ischemic Activity in Patients with Ischemic Heart Disease." *American Heart Journal.* July 2003; 146: 55-61.

Joliffe et al., *Chochrane Database.* Syst. Rev. 2001.

Jorenby et al., "A Controlled Trial of Sustained-Release Bupropion, a Nicotine Patch, or Both for Smoking Cessation." *New England Journal of Medicine.* Mar. 4, 1999; 340: 685-91.

Kawachi, I, D Sparrow et al., "A Prospective Study of Anger and Coronary Heart Disease: The Normative Aging Study." *Circulation.* Nov. 1, 1996; 94: 2090-95.

Ko et al., "Beta-Blocker Therapy and Symptoms of Depression, Fatigue, and Sexual Dysfunction." *Journal of the American Medical Association.* 2002; 288: 351-7.

Lesperance et al., "Depression and 1-Year Prognosis in Unstable Angina." *Archives of Internal Medicine*. May 8, 2000; 160: 1354-60.

Levin et al., "Cardiac Rehabilitation—a Cost Analysis." *Journal of Internal Medicine*. 1991; 230: 427-434.

Nickolaus, M et al., "Advances in Interventional Cardiology." *Nursing Clinics of North America*. Dec. 2000; 35(4): 897-912.

National Heart, Lung and Blood Institute. *Morbidity and Mortality: 1998 chartbook on cardiovascular, Lung and Blood Diseases*. Rockville, MD: US Deptartment of Health and Human Services, National Institutes of Health, 1998.

McGovern, P, D Jacobs Jr. et al., "The Minnesota Heart Survey. Trends in Acute Coronary Heart Disease Mortality, Morbidity, and Medical Care from 1985 through 1997." *Circulation*. July, 2001; 104: 19-24.

MacMahon, et al., "Blood Pressure, Stroke, and Coronary Heart Disease." *The Lancet*. March 31, 1990; 335: 765-74.

Milani et al., "Effects of Cardiac Rehabilitation and Exercise Training Programs on Depression in Patients after Major Coronary Events." *American Heart Journal*. 1996; 132: 726-32.

Mittleman, et al., "Educational Attainment, Anger, and the Risk for Triggering Myocardial Infarction Onset. The Determinants of Myocardial Infarction Onset Study Investigators." *Archives of Internal Medicine*. Apr. 14, 1997; 157: 769-775.

O'Connor et al., "An Overview of Randomized Trials of Rehabilitation with Exercise after Myocardial Infarction." *Circulation*. 1989; 80: 234-244.

Post Coronary Artery Bypass Graft Trial Investigators, The, "Effects of Treating Depression and Low Perceived Social Support on Clinical Events After Myocardial Infarction." *Journal of the American Medical Association*. June 18, 2003; 289: 3106-16.

Prabhakar et al., "The Risks of Moderate and Extreme Obesity for Coronary Artery Bypass Grafting Outcomes: A Study from the Society of Thoracic Surgeons' Database." *Annals of Thoracic Surgery*. 2002; 74: 1125-31.

"Randomized Trial of Cholesterol Lowering in 4444 Patients with Coronary Heart Disease: The Scandinavian Simvastatin Survival Study (4S)." *The Lancet*. Nov. 19, 1994; 344(8934): 1383-9.

Rea et al., "Smoking Status and Risk for Recurrent Coronary Events after Myocardial Infarction." *Annals of Internal Medicine*. Sept. 17, 2002; 137(6):494-500.

Rivers et al., "Reinfarction after Thrombolytic Therapy for Acute Myocardial Infarction Followed by Conservative Management: Incidence and Effect of Smoking." *Journal of the American College of Cardiology*. Aug. 1990; 16: 340-8.

Rosenberg et al., "The Risk of Myocardial Infarction after Quitting Smoking in Men Under 55 Years of Age." *New England Journal of Medicine*. Dec. 12, 1985; 313: 1511-4.

Rosenberg et al. "Decline in the Risk of Myocardial Infarction Among Women Who Stop Smoking." *New England Journal of Medicine*. Jan. 25, 1990; 322: 213-7.

Sacks et al. "The Effect of Pravastatin on Coronary Events after Myocardial Infarction in Patients with Average Cholesterol Levels." *New England Journal of Medicine*. Oct. 3, 1996; 335: 1001-9.

Schwann et al., "Effects of Body Size on Operative, Intermediate and Long-Term Outcomes after Coronary Artery Bypass Operation." *Annals of Thoracic Surgery*. 2001; 71: 521-31.

Stamler et al., "Is Relationship Between Serum Cholesterol and Risk of Premature Death from Coronary Heart Disease Continuous and Graded?" *Journal of the American Medical Association*. Nov. 1986; 256: 2823-28.

Todd et al., "Effect of Exercise Training on the Total Ischaemic Burden: an Assessment by 24 hour Ambulatory Electrocardiographic Monitoring." *British Heart Journal*. 1992; 68: 560-6.

Watkins et al., "Cognitive and Somatic Symptoms of Depression are Associated with Medical Comorbidity in Patients after Acute Myocardial Infarction." *American Heart Journal*. July 2003; 146: 48-54.

Weisman et al., "Evaluation of the Benefits and Risks of Low-Dose Aspirin in the Secondary Prevention of Cardiovascular and Cerebrovascular Events." *Archives of Internal Medicine*. Oct. 28, 2002; 162: 2197-202.

Williams et al., "Early Exercise Training in Patients Older than Age 65 Years Compared with that in Younger Patients after Acute Myocardial Infarction or Coronary Atery Bypass Grafting." *American Journal of Cardiology*. 1985; 55: 263-6.

Willich et al., "Association of Wake Time and the Onset of Myocardial Infarction." *Circulation*. Dec. 1991; 84[suppl VI]: 62-7.

Index

♦ ♦ ❖ ♦ ♦ ♦ ❖ ♦ ♦ ♦ ❖ ♦ ♦ ♦ ❖ ♦ ♦ ♦ ❖ ♦ ♦

ELECTROCARDIOGRAM, 290

ELECTROLYTES, 290

EMERGENCY ROOM,
ADVANCEMENTS IN THE, 43–44

EMOTIONS AND YOUR HEALTH,
LINK BETWEEN, 254–255

ENDOTHELIAL CELLS, 290

EPINEPHRINE, 290

EXERCISE, 160–161, 161–168.
SEE ALSO CARDIAC
REHABILITATION

AND BETA-BLOCKERS, 172–173

AND EMOTIONAL LEVELS,
163–164

AND HEART FUNCTION,
164–165

AND HOSPITALIZATION,
161–162

AND OLDER PATIENTS, 169

AND RECOVERY, 162–163

AND SURVIVAL RATES, 160–161

AND THE ARTERIES, 172

AND THE DAMAGED HEART, 170

AND THE HEART MUSCLE,
170–171

BENEFITS OF, 166–167

F

FAMILY, ROLE OF THE, 32

FAT, 290

FATIGUE, 24, 25

FIBRIC ACID DERIVATIVES, 282,
290

FIBRILLATION, 290

FIGHT OR FLIGHT RESPONSE,
103–104

FOAM CELLS, 52, 290

FORSSMANN, WERNER, 42

FRAMINGHAM HEART STUDY, 290

FRIEDBERG, CHARLES K., 36, 38,
40

G

GLOMERULUS, 290

GLUCOSE, 290

GLYCEMIC INDEX, 290

GLYCOSYLATED HEMOGLOBIN
(HBAC) LEVELS, 290

GRUENZIG, ANDREAS, 42

H

HEART

CALCULATION OF HEART RATE,
50

OXYGEN SUPPLY, 48–49

REQUIREMENTS OF, 50–51

STRUCTURE, 47

HEART ATTACK, 8, 21–22, 28,
63–64

HEART BLOCK, 290